Get

Smarter

Keys to Improving Brain Function

(Increase Your Intelligence and Become the Greatest Version of Yourself)

Stanley Fleming

Published By **Regina Loviusher**

Stanley Fleming

*Get Smarter: Keys to Improving Brain Function
(Increase Your Intelligence and Become the
Greatest Version of Yourself)*

ISBN   978-1-7776534-8-4

Legal & Disclaimer

The information contained in this book is not designed to replace or take the place of any form of medicine or professional medical advice. The information in this book has been provided for educational & entertainment purposes only.

The information contained in this book has been compiled from sources deemed reliable, and it is accurate to the best of the Author's knowledge; however, the Author cannot guarantee its accuracy and validity and cannot be held liable for any errors or omissions. Changes are periodically made to this book. You must consult your doctor or get professional medical advice before using any of the suggested remedies, techniques, or information in this book.

Upon using the information contained in this book, you agree to hold harmless the Author from and against any damages, costs, and expenses, including any legal fees potentially resulting from the application of any of the information provided by this guide. This disclaimer applies to any damages or injury caused by the use and application, whether directly or indirectly, of any advice or information presented, whether for breach of contract, tort, negligence, personal injury, criminal intent, or under any other cause of action.

You agree to accept all risks of using the information presented inside this book. You need to consult a professional medical practitioner in order to ensure you are both able and healthy enough to participate in this program.

Table Of Contents

Chapter 1: Dialogue and Common Grammar Mistakes

Numerous words individuals mix up while talking and writing. In conversations, essays an email, a letter or even in a Facebook status. You're bound to make yourself look foolish. You must take your time to comprehend the meaning behind what you're writing or saying and make sure you do it right. The truth is that English is the most challenging spoken language around the globe, but it's not a reason to not learn the language. It's astonishing how many of the most basic English words are misused and mispelled on a regular routine. Make sure to clarify any word is used, otherwise you're likely to end up being snubbed eventually. A lot of what I've written in the beginning will to be so straightforward it's easy to think that I'm being condescending But I'm not. Many people commit even the simplest of errors in their language. What's important is to identify your mistakes and fixing the problem as soon as you can, since small mistakes can make you appear stupid, believe me. Don't be offended by the way basic the basic information. Be aware that I wrote this guide for as broad an audience as I can, and that we must start by learning the basics before we can move forward.

1.) Beware of those who confuse basic terms like then vs. It's amazing the amount of times this specific scenario is brought up. It's true that if I'm looking through an applicant's resume to my clinic and notice a few grammatical errors like these (it is a common occurrence all the time) My evaluation of this person's suitability to be a good fit for the position drops substantially. When you're comparing two items you should use more than. For instance: I prefer these shoes over the other shoes. If you're discussing things that took place during a specific time or for a term that's basically interchangeable with then, choose then. Then, when I was younger, I was an entirely different individual. Ex: I'd like to visit the mall first, then to go to the water park. One trick for remembering this is"I would use the word"then" instead of then, however afterward I got better than what I had been. If you're having difficulty recalling the correct word to use, just repeat the following small sentence over and over again and you'll be capable of figuring it out.

2) SAW VS SEEN. It's a nagging one as I hear it all everyday. It seems that Canadians struggle more in this regard more than Americans. SAW can be used in the past present. For instance, I watched the exact same film this week. The word "sEEN" is usually employed in conjunction with words have, had been, are, or were.

For instance: Mary had seen Joe twice over the course of her last year. In 5th grade, I can remember that there was an elementary school girl known as Jill who was constantly referring to the term "seen," and this drove me mad. Her mantra was always "Yea but I've already had that experience before." Be careful not to be Jill. There's a method to recall"She was there, however, Steve was able to see it years back.'

3) ACCEPT VS EXCEPT. It's another of my least favorite words in this article. The word "except" can be used to replace the word Other than. Ex: I enjoyed everything about the meal, with the exception for soup. ACCEPT can be used in the event that you're receiving some kind of. Ex: I've agreed to the conditions and terms of the contract. There's a method to remember"I acknowledge the word accept, notwithstanding where it's misused.'

4) AFFECT VS EFFECT. It is a problem for me and I also mix up these terms often time. AFFECT is the word used to describe the power of alter. Ex: The latest information definitely influenced the professor's choice. EFFECT refers to the effect or consequence. Ex: The impact on these changes are intense. This is a trick I employ: "The winds impacted my hair however, it did not have any impact on the hair of Linda.'

5) IGNORANT. The word "IGNORANT" doesn't convey rudeness or demeaning. It is a sign of lack of knowledge of general knowledge or education. For instance, sometimes being ignorant is the most effective way to stay happy. That is the reason they say that ignorance is bliss.

6) WHICH VS WITCH. It's a much less frequent error, yet I frequently see it. It is utilized when seeking specific data out of a specific set or in the case of referencing an

item that has already been mentioned. For example: Which of these options is your preferred choice? WITCH is definitely a sinister ugly, ugly woman with the Broomstick. The most wellknown method I've seen people employ"Who is which witch is it?'

7.) A broader vocabulary can be a guaranteed approach to influence positively how people view you. Another way to broaden your vocabulary is by signing to receive a 'word for the day' at Dictionary.com. Each day, you'll get an email detailing a word along with its definition. There are times when these terms don't seem to be relevant to the real world at all, but occasionally you will discover a word you could quickly incorporate into your daily vocabulary. If you're trying to look an oldfashioned person, then just flip the dictionary and open a random page and choose a term you'd like to know.

8.) When you're reading when you stumble upon a term you do not comprehend, don't avoid the word. Find the word immediately before rereading the passage you came across the word within so that you are able to comprehend it within the context of. I have found that searching for words in an oldfashioned dictionary to be superior tool over searching it on Google. If you search for a word in a dictionary, you need to put some effort, which means that once you have found the meaning, you're much likely to be able to remember the word because you have to search for it. When you press a button and locate the word on the internet, there's virtually no effort required. I've noticed that I don't remember the meaning in a matter of minutes which is why I have to google every word I come across.

9.) Here are a few fantastic phrases you could immediately begin making use of that show you're armed with a smart arsenal of terms in your vocabulary:

Epitome: The ideal instance of something. "He was the epitome the best sportsman.'

Accolade is a tangible signification or reward in recognition of something. The accolades that came with a successful musical career are evident.'

Quintessential: The most common example of something. She was the perfect excellent girl.

Zenith: The topmost spot. It is the time that something is the most effective or efficient. The basketball soared to its highest point up in the air, and fell smoothly onto the ground.'

Audacity: The willingness to take risks that are risky. "She was brave enough to request that the company cover her travel expenses.'

Esoteric is intended for understanding by only a tiny number of individuals."The professor's esoteric philosophical lecture was difficult to comprehend.

Euphemism for "to sugar wrap' or coat something in order to give it a more appealing sound than what it really is. In lieu of telling him that he had been fired The boss took an euphemism to say he was letting go.

Verbose means using many words that are not needed. "My boss rambled for 15 minutes in a very in a ranting manner.'

Incessant: Continuously going on with no pause, hesitation, or hesitation. "The waves repeatedly crashed into the shoreline.

Splice: Join, or join. A bungee cord was tied on the last side of the hammock.'

Freudian Slip: An error made during a conversation that may be a sign of an unconsciously idea, belief, or emotional state. "She said she hated his mother. She says she intended to be brother. He believes she might have made the Freudian slip.

Faux Pas: An embarrassing act in a social situation. Steve committed an error by walking into an outdoor pool, while looking at the woman.'

The Nirvana, a paradise that is a place of total peace and joy. "Hawaii" is a form of nirvana designed for surfers who are extreme.'

Narcissist is someone who is completely obsessive about their own selfimage. The woman stares at her mirror for greater portion of an hour each morning. This is the way I am sure she is an Narcissist.'

Verbatim: A term to word copies. "Her notes were verbatim copies of her notes on the whiteboard.'

Suave: charming and chic. His suave manner of speaking was enticing to women who were present in the space.'

Malleable: Easy to influence or altered. "His mind was as malleable and flexible as hot metal in the blacksmith's shop.'

Chagrin: Embarrassment. To my dismay, I was not chosen to take part in the contest.'

Extremely excited. "Paul might perhaps have been overconfident regarding his interview.'

Vicarious: Experienced by someone else. "When I watch hockey, I am able to feel as if I'm as a player.'

Voracious means eating the best features of the thing. "The black hole was an enormous maw that devoured all that it came across and even the light.'

Inconspicuous: Minimal and not worth noticing. "A car that doesn't have a exhaust is the exact opposite of anything that's unnoticed.'

Liability is the act of being responsible for an event or. "She was a public risk because she drove having a broken arm.'

Crux: The main problem, the essence of an item. The crux of the case of murder was definitely the knife that was bloody.'

Veracity: Habitual truthfulness. He gave ample evidence to believe that he demonstrated high veracity with his honest responses.'

10.) If you play scrabble, you'll be able to increase your vocabulary rapidly If you're not afraid of embarrassing your pals. Being a seasoned scrabble player, I'll give you a few suggestions on how you can play very well at the game to ensure that the the next time you play, you'll have everyone awestruck.

There is no place in the scrabble rulesbook is it stated that you have to be aware of the precise meaning of each word you type. This makes scrabble a challenge for professionals. That means if you're able to remember words regardless of whether you understand the word that you could become an extremely dangerous weapon in scrabble. It is true that scrabble is a test with current knowledge about words however it's an opportunity to learn to expand your vocabulary.

Two letter words are considered to be the most holy of scrabble as they permit players to join words would otherwise be impossible. Also, to the surprise of many, turn out to be one of the most rewarding terms in the game provided you're playing them correctly. If you can master these, you'll almost be the best at scrabble. Below are the complete list of twoletter scrabble terms and a lot of them are not been aware of:

AA, AB, AD, AE, AG, AH, AI, AL, AM, AN, AR, AS, AT, AW, AX, AY, BA, BE, BI, BO BY, CH, DA, DE, DI, DO, EA, ED, EE, EF, EH, EL, EM, EN, ER, ES, ET, EX, FA, FE, FY, GI, GO, GU, HA, HE, HI, HM, HO, ID, IF, IN, IO, IS, IT, JA, JO, KA, KI, KO, KY, LA, LI, LO, MA, ME, MI, MM, MO, MU, MY, NA, NE, NO, NU, NY, OB, OD, OE, OF, OH, OI, OM, ON, OO, OP, OR, OS, OU, OW, OX, OY, PA, PE, PI, PO, QI, RE, SH, SI, SO, ST, TA, TE, TI, TO, UG, UH, UM, UN, UP, UR, US, UT, WE, WO, XI, XU, YA, YE, YO, YU, ZA, ZO.

Words QI as well as ZA have been the winners in many more scrabble contests than I know how many, mostly because I put them on tripleletter score tiles. A lot of people are shocked to realize that IM isn't a 2letter scrabble word. This is because IM is an abbreviation that isn't allowed in scrabble. Do you understand what I'm trying to say?

11) Every day you read is an excellent opportunity to acquire vocabulary. These are a few books I strongly suggest to anyone: The Rise of Superman The 4Hour Body The 4% Universe, Cosmos, Death by Black Hole, Into the Wild, Paddle to the Amazon, The Hobbit, Life of Pi, Rich Dad Poor Dad, Rich Dad's The Guide to investing, A Painted House, The Great Gatsby and of obviously The Dictionary! I enjoy reading novels, but I have found reading nonfiction books to prove to be more beneficial and practical. The ability to imagine is always enjoyable, but getting realworld information is the most beneficial, for me.

12) Be the best friend you can with A Thesaurus. Learning to use words in a variety of ways will help your mind to not be repetitious when you talk and write. This will likewise increase the vocabulary of your.

13) Maybe I went through an unrelated midlife crises a couple of years ago however, I was really interested in rap music. It just seemed foreign to my eardrums that I fell in love instantly. The focus wasn't on beats, or even the precise purpose of the track. The thing that intrigued me was how the artists were able to melt English language until it was so flexible that they were able to manipulate it in any way they liked. Every song turned into a puzzle that I tried to unravel. I was interested in knowing what the musicians could do to fit phrases where they seemed to not be. I also discovered a lot of new words from

watching rap music, and particularly, Eminem. In no way am I accepting the homophobic or misogynistic lyrics of the man. It is essential to recognize that he's one of the most acclaimed poets to have ever lived on this earth. There's been no better writer. Also that if you are listening to some Eminem tracks, you'll be able to learn a variety of terms that you did not even realize existed.

14) If you are learning an unfamiliar word, you should instantly incorporate it into a everyday conversation. It's all about practice, however make sure you start slowly. If you're contemplating making a speech in public using lots of words aren't wellknown to you it might be time to consider rethinking your decision. As you've probably guessed that nobody is more stupid when they're caught making use of a term (besides the scrabble) which

they don't understand the meaning behind.

*BONUS TIP # 2

Beware of stall terms at all at all costs! Stall words are phrase like the word "um, ah," you know, or (the less appropriate word) fu*#ing. Avoid filling in gaps in your conversation by using stall terms that are short particularly with the term fu*#ing. This isn't a joke and all too often hear the following example: "Man fu*#ing Chris the yesterday, would you like to find out what he did? The guy says the man is thinking of selling the gorgeous lakefront home!"

They appear as if you are unable to think clearly and definitely seem less wise. My wife says the word "like" far often and I'm trying to persuade her to quit. I too am frequently guilty of using the word "umm". Although I'm getting better at it but I must focus on securing my words. You should take your time to talk slowly and clearly; it's acceptable to pause for a few seconds during your conversation. If you're visiting someone who is meeting for the first time make sure you give them a solid handshake. ensure that you are in contact with them at all moments and avoid using techniques that make you sound like a staller. Slowly, clearly and clearly If you want to grab the attention of someone. The use of slack words makes you look unfocused, and a smooth voice can make you appear knowledgeable and intelligent.

Chapter 2: Question Everything

15) Guilt and pure skepticism both fall on opposite sides in the spectrum. It is best to aim for somewhere in between for people who want to believe in your argument. A person who is skeptical of any information regardless of contradictory evidence, is thought to be irrational and stupid. In contrast anyone who is deceived and trusts everything they read can be deemed weakminded and insular. Be logical in deciding which to believe or not that something. Think about whether you are bias or do you believe that the source of information is bias and is the source trustworthy is it trustworthy, and does the source hold the right to influence people to believe in a certain item, and have you analyzed each side of the story. After you've answered each of these questions it is time to think critically about the information that you're likely to accept as fact. Keep in mind that doubting anything

doesn't make you smart! In reality, it makes appear like one of the pompous types.

16) It's not possible to define a concept as a dumb inquiry, until you pose an unintelligible question. It's true that there's a phenomenon known called the fabled "dumb question. The term "dumb question" can be posed when you speak prior to thinking. When asking a question you must take a moment to consider your knowledge already. Consider the query several times and you may be able to generate answers. Naturally, there will be times when there is a legitimate reason to not know the right answer (unless of course you're a kind or god. If you're absolutely unable to find what the answer is and you've attempted to think of your own answer best guess, always pose a question rather than think you've got the

answer. Everyone hates a bullshitter particularly a bad one.

In some instances, if you're in the course of a conversation, and someone mentions an expression, a phrase or an item of information that which you do not understand you may be able to go on and pretend that you are aware of what's being discussed. DON'T DO THIS. It's better to be educated and be a bit naive rather than remain in ignorance. Questioning is the only method of learning as humans And if you're asking questions, you have everything you need to know. Because the former is impractical, you should be curious.

17) Engage with and inquire about individuals from every walk of life. Sometimes the most powerful solutions will come from most unlikely people. It's not my intention to dwell on my journey to Brazil however, just before meeting

Raiza I was introduced to an elderly gentleman known as Phillipe. Phillipe was extremely poor, and also a resident of the favelas. I offered him money in case he ran out on the street. He was grateful and then went with me for time. I inquired about his goals and hopes would be for the coming years. The answer I received still amazes me. He told me "My fantasies? In all likelihood, I may be in the middle of thinking about them right now. The world I live in could seem so dull and perfect, that I've constructed a lengthy, challenging vision that I have to work through. If I do experience a similar issue in real day life, I'll have the knowledge to tackle the issue. If this is indeed the case and my life seems to be perfect but dull and monotonous and predictable, it's best to remain here.

Chapter 3: Remember, Remember

18) Memory I believe that memory is the core of intelligence. Imagine if you could flawlessly remember every bit of information your brain was exposed to. It would be incomparably skilled. We're not saying that you require a flawless memory, but enhancing your capacity to remember lots of facts immediately is extremely essential. A reason that people seek to increase their memory in order to recognize names of acquaintances when they meet them. There's not a single thing to be more embarrassing than waking up to realize that you don't know what they're called. One trick I employ to remember people's names is to repeat their name. After meeting someone, you must keep using the name of that person as you talk with them. This doesn't need to be bizarre. Here's an example of how to:

Theo"Theo "I'm Theo, pleased to meet you."

Jack"Jack "Hello My Name is Jack."

Theo"Theo "Where is your home? Jack?"

Jack"Jack" St Louis, what do you think of yourself?"

Theo"I'm originally from B.C., Canada. Why did you decide to move here to Chicago?"

Jack"Business normal, how is your opinion?"

Theo"Theo" Jack, I don't not want to even consider the word "business" tonight. This has consumed my entire life."

JackJack" You're right, that's a good idea. Now I need to go I enjoyed meeting you. Sorry to bother you, but what did you mean when you told me what your name was?"

TheoTheo" It's not necessary to apologize. It's Theo. Thank you for your time. Jack I had pleasure to have met you."

It's as easy as it gets. Like I said, it does not have to be a snarky thing. It's just a matter of repeating the name of your loved one a couple of times to effectively associate their image and their name. If you follow this method, I can assure you that you won't ever forget a name.

19) Get your brain working! Just like I stated previously, your brain functions as a muscle, and must be kept in good shape. One of my preferred methods to exercise my brain is playing the game of chess. Chess is an extremely physically demanding game. For a player to be successful, you need to be unpredictable. However, you must also be able to anticipate the moves of your opponent. Strategize and be adept at attacking, but you also need to know how you need to

defend. Check out several YouTube videos, master the basics of strategies, and do a lot of practice then you'll soon enjoy the satisfying sensation of winning chess tournaments.

20) Engage in additional brainbased activities. Try the Sudoku puzzle once or twice every week. You can also join the renowned website 'Lumosity as well as develop an individual training plan. A great challenge for your mind is solving crossword puzzles. These puzzles can stretch your mind to the limits and I would highly recommend them to anyone. Even though they are sometimes frustrating, I believe they're extremely helpful. They'll increase the vocabulary of your brain and help you remember information better (words).

21) I'm not planning to appear like the saints. When I was younger, I was a smoker. It may seem strange to be

discussing the effects of a substance that could adversely affect memory in a chapter on memory, but let me to clarify. The majority of evidence on marijuana and loss of shortterm memory is not conclusive. It's not as if I'm encouraging you to get out and get high, attempt to recall some important information. It's not like it's a good idea for everybody. My request is that you get rid of any stigma that marijuana has briefly, pause your thoughts and take a look. It is just the plant. It is not my experience to smoke marijuana in order to ease pain or cope anxiety. If people are using it to relieve stress or pain, they're more likely to develop an addiction to the drug. In fact, contrary what is popular, one could become addicted to marijuana. In fact, you could become addicted to everything: yoga, video games TV, political reading, and the possibilities are endless.

If something isn't in line with to the standard medical definition of physical addiction, it may remain an addiction. In my case, as I've said before I've didn't use marijuana for the purpose of overcoming any issue, but I did use it to aid in the process of thinking and an experiment in the sense that you can call it an experiment. If you're not aware that there are two varieties of marijuana, indica, which can give you the drowsy, relaxing effect and sativa, that gives the user a lively, brain racing buzz. I smoked in the second. Marijuana can truly open the mind to new realms of thought that were prior to now. Any thing that triggers amazing and often new thoughts shouldn't be dismissed as a flimsy idea. There are times when use marijuana, there's very little or nothing to gain, and what you get is a few snarky conversations with acquaintances, but we're not discussing these times. We're talking about times where marijuana has the power to permanently change the way you think in positive ways. The occasions when it will help to discover the most intimate functions of your brain and the occasions when marijuana can help you be more compassionate towards other people, and the occasions when it may trigger fresh and inspiring thoughts, those times when it has the power to scare your mind enough to make you humble and transform you into a comfortable, relaxed human being. Nature provides us with something that is able to significantly impact the entire world.

Marijuana has been legalized rapidly throughout North America. Is it occurring without reason? The main chemical present found in cannabis, THC, can be employed to sleep aid, to provide the relief of pain and to help people struggling with emotional and mental traumas like

PTSD. As with all substances, marijuana may be misused and used in excess however if you manage to achieve a healthy balance it can alter how you view your world. I've experienced countless positive outcomes from marijuana, I don't have any doubt that the plant has helped me become a more conscious, selfaware and reflective person. If it doesn't mean that I'm smarter because of it and more aware, I'm not sure the reason why. If you're concerned about the damage to your lungs, then smoking vaporizers is your ideal choice. The worldrenowned astronomer, scientist, cosmologist, astrophysicist and writer Carl Sagan has been quoted as in a statement, "The illegality of cannabis is shocking, and a hindrance in the full use of a substance that helps to bring peace, insight as well as the sensitivity and friendship which are desperately required in our everincreasingly dangerous and chaotic world."

22) Tim Ferris discusses in his book "The 4Hour Body,"" an event Tim Ferris attended along with Richard Branson (Founder of Virgin Group Net Worth = 4.9 billion) In the meeting, Branson was asked to be more productive. Branson was contemplating briefly before he replied "workout." Training will help lower stress levels, boost the energy level of our day and, ultimately, we become more efficient people. I've recently begun doing a few exercises a day but it was difficult to settle into an established routine. After I got in routine I was able to see the increase in my productivity. Branson did not lie. The tiniest eBook I downloaded recently on Amazon named "Health and Fitness from Scratch" written by John Mayo, helped me to follow a detailed workout program that is suitable for novices. The author also

includes his email address within the book, so that if I wanted to know more, I could contact directly. I thought that this was a great idea therefore I've also included my email address towards the conclusion of the book.

23) Be in 'the zone' more frequently. It's true that 'the zone' or the flow state according to "The The Rise of Superman" by Steven Kotler is a real and real thing. To be able to reach the maximum potential of humans, it is necessary to discover the mysteries of flow. In the way that Kotler says, if we place ourselves in risky situations such as skydiving and diving into deep water, rock climbing racing or diving There is a dramatic change. Focus increases and we are able to lose any sense of selfconsciousness. time is altered and seems to be slowing down and we get absorbed by the activities. In this time the brain gets filled with dopamine that

increases our attention, information movement, patterns of recognition the rate of blood flow and firing time. Also, we get an injection of Norepinephrine that increases respiration speed and stimulates the release of glucose in order to provide our bodies with energy. Also, endorphins release which ease discomfort and provide satisfaction. Anandamide, an endogenous neurotransmitter that is produced by the body increases our mood, reduces our anxiety and allows our brains to think laterally. It also plays an important role in the high we experience after smoking marijuana. The last neurochemical released is once the flow state has been achieved and it is called seratonin. It aids people in coping with stress and remain in a healthy state of mind.

A flow state isn't as intense as an adrenaline rush! The stress response is adrenaline (fight or fight) in which the brain shifts to a survival mode. A state of flow is a state of problemsolving which allows your brain think rationally through a problem and handle the situation on the spot in real time. That doesn't mean that you must turn into an extreme sport addict If you're competent enough to tap into this state of mind however, putting yourself in a challenging circumstances every now and then and you are able to overcome it, you won't regret doing it. I've been doing skydiving since the age of 11. I'll never forget that first time I fell from an aircraft in the air at an altitude of 10,000 feet. I felt all of the listed signs of being in a state of flow, and the aweinspiring high. Once I was home the world seemed to be completely different. It was like my brain processes had gone to such a high level that they became extended and reenforced. I was able be more clear and rationally. Conversations seemed more fluid and my speech were more refined. I was hooked on this zone, and kept jumping in the sky to gain access to it on a regular basis.

24) Visualize every single thing! The potential of visualisation is amazing. Every time many people believe an action to be impossible until they observe others do it. If we observe someone doing something, we're able to envision ourselves doing it making it easy. This is especially true when you're the first person to perform something however. I can remember seeing Travis Pastrana do the first back flip he did on his dirt bicycle. It must be that he had an extremely strong mental psyche that allowed him to envision him doing something that, at the time was considered to be unattainable. Back flips have now been a common trick for dirt bike races and a double flip has been done.

Kotler further describes a twelveweek study, where participants tried to build strength in the muscles of their fingers and arms. The group that engaged their arms and fingers saw most significant increases in strength. However, the test group that did intense visualization exercises but did not actually engage in exercise at all, experienced the strength gain by 35% on their fingers, and 13.5 percentage for their arms. This is a clear indication that visualization can be a tool which works, and it does so effectively. The majority of people don't advise you to "sleep" on your issues to aren't thinking about these issues. This is to help you better imagine a situation and tackle it the right manner. When the next time you face a difficult job to finish, such as the job interview, examination, or competition You should imagine the job and visualize yourself doing precisely the way you would like to.

It may sound absurd, but it actually can be very effective.

25) Take a large amount of brainfriendly foods! What do you think it will take for your brain to operate in a way that is optimal in the absence of providing your brain with enough energy and nutrition? The foods I like the most for my brain are kale, spinach and eggs, as well as fish and broccoli. I also love blueberries, pumpkin seeds almonds, chia seeds citrus fruits, kiwi, sage and bananas. I also take vitamin B12 (for blood circulation and brain function) as well as an Omega 3 fish oil pill (to reduce triglyceride levels and assist in joint lubrication, and to prevent cognitive decline) each morning.

Chapter 4: Passion Knowledge

26) I am fascinated by people who love something and even subjects that I don't have any interest in. How people get fascinated by certain topics is always fascinating to me. This is among the main reasons that led me to pursue a career as psychologist so I can better understand the causes of obsession. It is evident that there are many unhealthy obsessives, but we're focused only on positive obsessions.

The best method to master the insides of something is to be enthralled by the subject. It will take your attention over time, until you're completely informed regarding the subject. I've always wished to repair my own vehicles, as automobiles have always fascinated me. I also wanted to cut costs on mechanics. I began studying automobiles and eventually my brain was occupied. I would practice getting different pieces of equipment out of my vehicle and then put them back into. I grew so familiar with automobiles that I could engage in deep conversations with fellow automobile enthusiasts and still not appear like a total moron. This was truly a wonderful experience and really demonstrated how well the passion of a person really can work.

If you're attracted to something, you should take time to take the time to be passionate about it to be more informed. As you develop more interests will make you more educated and knowledgeable will be. Even if others don't have the same passions as you but they'll surely be impressed by what you've learned and see your self as more knowledgeable.

*BONUS TIP # 3

True, the perception of intelligence is crucial, however at the time you will know if you're just a great faker. Don't stop in your pursuit of knowledge! The more you learn you know, the more people be able to respect what you communicate (if you've completed the right homework). When you first wake up, you can try hopping on your laptop and browsing until you find something interesting. Be sure to really master this, however. It is my experience that having the endless information available on the Internet often makes me feel smug as I know that should I don't remember information, I will instantly find it. But, when you are in a discussion, you don't want to be the person that always checks their smartphone for confirmation. It is better to understand the details well.

Look the Part

27) 27) You do not need to own a lavish wardrobe of designer brands like Lacoste, Hugo Boss and Ralph Lauren. However, what you need to remember is that the

clothes you put on and the way in which you look after your body directly affects how others will view your appearance. People can be very critical and look for every reason to discredit the things you say to them.

I can remember when I was in high school one of my buddies from an alternative school was always fond of to dress in baggy clothes. On Halloween, in the year 11 we decided to change our clothes. I was wearing one of his oversized sweaters as well as an untight pair of jeans while he was wearing one of my polo's that fit along with my finest jeans. The experience for me was not the best, in part because I was invisible. Everyone knew it was Halloween but no one really paid any attention to the fact that I wore costumes, and they believed that I was an fool. For one of my friends, the incident was "mindblowing." It was the sole black student at school wearing clothes like that. The person I spoke to said that they liked him, his they listened to him, and he felt valued. He told me that he was able to observe the different between people's eyes. They were receptive to what he had speak and considered him to be someone on the same level of intelligence. He was not even aware his costume to celebrate Halloween. In fact, He believes that no one even noticed him up until the day. Following that the man went to a store to buy some new clothes. It wasn't expensive, but an polo shirt, pair of dress shirts as well as a pair of dark, fitted jeans. As I mentioned, this does not have to be an expense You just need be willing to put a time and effort into be sure that you're looking like someone who is a shrewd and intelligent person.

28) You should surround yourself with positive smart individuals. If you are

surrounded by drunken people constantly time there's a good chance... it's because you're an idiot who is drunk. It is important to ensure that you are surrounded by people who test you and force you to think regularly. Engaging in conversations which you're fully involved in is a crucial element of growing into a more intelligent person. It's not that I'm saying people should surround themselves with pompous experts. It is important to find individuals who are downto the earth, friendly and at ease with who they're. There's nothing more frustrating than someone trying to hide their anxieties by trying to look smart. People like this were throughout my philosophy classes at the University, which made me nauseous! Anyone who doesn't think they are competent to be learning. If you're incapable of learning, it is a sign that you aren't clever.

Also, you should seek out great role models and teachers. You should find someone who is superior, smarter, and more intelligent than you are try to emulate the person. The way you think about intelligence, just like anything that is in this world is completely dependent. It's possible that you're the most intelligent person in your area and yet there's an area a couple of miles away, and there's a person who in that town is two times more intelligent than you are you clever in comparison? Choose mentors/ role models you believe as being relatively smart compared with world population.

Chapter 5: Stay Current

29) Being aware of the current events around the globe is an excellent way to improve your general intelligence. Engaging in dialogues about global issues can be a profound knowledge experience. There's a chance to get newspapers if you're in the old high school, or go to the Internet. My preferred source for news and, according to me, the most trustworthy is VICE News. VICE's CEO VICE is Shane Smith, and this man is a pro. If he isn't sure of the subject and needs to know, that he researches the issue and then shares it with everyone in an impartial and transparent manner. The journalist goes to the deepest trenches in order to provide people with engaging and eyeopening news reports. The year 2008 was the time Shane Smith, a team comprised of VICE photographers and journalists traveled to North Korea. It was among the most intriguing news articles

I've ever seen, and I strongly recommend you go to YouTube and taking a look.

The fascinating news articles that are featured on VICE are innumerable and I recommend getting familiar with it to ensure that you can keep uptodate with current events all over the globe.

30) Discover random facts. Learning trivial details across a range of areas is always beneficial. Be sure, however, you're learning facts, you study them thoroughly. Fact implied an absolute truth. But with the advent of the Internet it is possible to find conflicting facts even for generally accepted information. There are many proofs for whatever you read about. There's nothing more embarrassing than having a disagreement with someone over things you don't have basis to back up. Simply because you've found someone's words convincing is not a guarantee that they are saying their statements true.

Don't learn a million random facts only to start spewing the information out like a dog that barks. No one likes a complete stranger, and so ensure that you don't become one. It has been my experience that those with the highest intelligence tend to be the least reserved. They do not have any proof, therefore they sit back until someone calls on their expertise, and then speak about what they've learned. That's the type of knowledgeable person you'd like to be.

Chapter 6: Your scientific step-by-step guide to becoming superhuman

Your body was made in order to guarantee the longevity of your species. Your body must live long enough in order to achieve that. To avoid using excessive energy, your body's main aim is to prevent dying. According to Asprey each cell of your body is specifically designed to perform as minimally as possible.He describes this as part of MeatOS which is your operating system for meat. The system operates behind the scenes and keeps you going through autopilot. It's similar to the operating system in the computer. If you take a shot of tequila The code instructs the liver to begin breaking down alcohol. The code also regulates your breathing, as well as blinking your eyes In the event that it's damaged and visible.

MeatOS could be targeted just like computers are able to be hacked in order to reach your goals faster. The strategy of smarter, not harder has its roots in this. Instead of letting your program take over your life, you're able the ability to control the code.

First, stop looking for short-term fixes and begin thinking about the long term. Stop your 30 days of rapid weight reduction plans and your most painful workout routines. Discover the shortcuts that will yield optimal results, and accept the sluggish side of you. To maximize the energy you have it is important to eat properly before you start thinking about hacking.

Asprey refers to the substances which hinder the absorption of minerals, vitamins as well as other nutrients in food items as antinutrients. they must be eliminated out of your diet. The author claims that phytic acids is the primary culprit. It is discovered in all kinds of processed meals made from plants and also in legumes, nuts, seeds and legumes, as well as all-grains, soy and even corn all of the foods which other people say are good for your health and our environment. Do not eat as many. What about the animal products? Asprey suggests staying clear of the factory-feeding of poultry, and limiting the consumption of pig products as well as avoiding alternatives to meat. Take fish moderately and well.Next take a look at whether you're receiving enough of the fat-soluble vitamins D A, K and E, as the majority of individuals who consume a diet that is regular aren't getting the proper amounts of these vitamins. Then, you can apply minerals in similar manner. The most important minerals are sodium, calcium, magnesium as well as potassium, the sulfate and phosphorus as well as iron. Additionally, trace elements such as Iodine, zinc, cobalt and copper are essential.

Doctor. Jordan Nguyen, a biomedical engineer, is attempting to make use of cutting-edge technology this 2-part series in order to realise a boy's greatest dreams. Jordan Nguyen has revealed to Riley Saban, 13, that he'll create an instrument that can allow Riley to achieve the unimaginable and might even be able to possess the ability to be a superhero. Will Riley change his mind to take advantage of Jordan's latest technology? Can Jordan's tech-driven dream become a reality? Will Riley become superpowerful?

Riley will be able to use "telekinetic control" which allows him to control technology throughout his surroundings in a non-physical method, in this instance through the eyes. He begins to work on an electronic headband that reacts to the movements of his eyes the electrical activity of his eyes in order to regulate lighting, as well as other household appliances remote.

The real goal of Riley's is to become the driver. To allow Riley to realize this dream, Jordan would have to make her do more. The new challenge is to Riley to be able to see the obstacles in the surrounding since Riley relies on his eyes via Jordan's headband. He will instead have develop his brain to depend on another sensor to direct him. It's a specific process referred to "spatial sensorial." Riley's vision is likely to replace by the sense of touch when the brain is trained to respond to the vibrations that come through sensors that are located on the car's exterior.

Riley has to commit lots of work for the technology to work. The eyes and the brain have to be taught to perform particular actions. Jordan as well as Riley each need to be successful in order to achieve this. Together, they show the amazing capabilities of the human brain utilized with technology that can enhance the brain's capabilities.

Jordan is expected to receive the support of experts in the field along the way. They'll help him achieve his bold goal, and will ask questions about Jordan's breakthroughs Are we more than we think to the day that technology can give our biological systems superhuman capabilities? What could the human body and mind evolve? How can the human brain become the most efficient computer despite the continuous advancements of technology?

Jordan and Riley have a huge job in front of them. Are they able to Riley help his brain make use of Jordan's tech? Is Jordan's tech-related dream coming real? When will Riley be able to become a superhero? Do you have any dreams that you wish you could be an superhero? The ability to do all tasks faster, better and with greater efficiency? The dream of yours is set becoming a reality, but! ChatGPT, the latest AI breakthrough, ChatGPT, can help to realize your potential, and improve the quality of your life. Learn about the ways ChatGPT could transform you a superhero will be discussed in this article and will include actual examples, humor as well as some scientific. Buckle to take a thrilling trip.

What is ChatGPT in The Birth of a Superhuman?

We'll begin by defining the meaning of ChatGPT is. ChatGPT is a model of language driven by AI which was developed by OpenAI in order to explain it into simple terms. It's principal goal is helping people like me and you to create text that is similar to human speech from input. However, that's just the top of the. ChatGPT is more than just a simple text generator. The limitless potential of your brain can be unleashed by it.

10 Ways ChatGPT Can Transform Your Life: Unleashing Your Superpowers

1. Developing Your Creativity

2. Are you struggling to write? The ability to think of ideas rapidly by using ChatGPT and turn you into an effective creative force. Choose a topic, and then watch it produces a flood of ideas.

3. Enhanced learning capabilities

4. The power of knowledge is in the mind, and ChatGPT lets you learn new things more efficiently than you have ever. It is able to summarize information or provide clarifications and even guide you through different fields. Let go of late-night research sessions, and welcome being able to learn new things every single time.

5. Excellent time management

6. It will be easy to feel speed-up power when you give tasks to ChatGPT. ChatGPT could help you complete more with less time in helping you compose emails as well as create social media posts, which allows you to focus on most important things.

7.A master of several languages

8. ChatGPT's features for translation allow users to communicate with people from around the world by removing the boundaries of language as well as making you an international citizen. You're now a powerful new superpower!

9. An increase in the emotional quotient

10. You are able to develop the ability to develop your emotional intelligence the ability of ChatGPT to assess emotions and provide emotional intelligent solutions. All over the world you'll create peace while

dealing with difficult social environments like a superhero.

Do not rely on the words we have to say. ChatGPT transforms lives by giving people benefits all across the globe. ChatGPT helps people becoming their superheroes in all aspects including successful businesspeople, to stressed parents. Are you still not convinced? Let's look at the ways ChatGPT can boost confidence in yourself and make you feel as super-human by helping you in routine assignments. If you're a student professional or seeking to improve your life, ChatGPT is here to assist you in every step of the way. You'll be amazed at the way more efficient efficient, productive, and successful your life becomes when you choose ChatGPT as your ally. Don't miss out on the opportunity to harness your power and enhance the tasks that you perform on a daily on a regular basis!

What exactly is biohacking in the first place? For those who aren't part of the biohacking world who have microchips implanted into their brains, fabricated eyes, etc this sounds like some kind of sci-fi-inspired cyborg idea that, for some, this is exactly what it is.

But for the normal ordinary person biohacking can refer to the use of any home remedy which can provide a significant benefit like the use of cold or heat treatments such as infrared saunas, intermittent fasting, incorporating the adaptogens and vitamins you need to your diet etc. You could have been biohacking in the past and not even realizing that you are doing it.

The most simple description is offered by self-help expert Tony Robbins and company: "Biohacking your body is about altering your embryology and enchantment with the help of science and experiments to boost energy and improve your energy levels." There are numerous opportunities for biohacking that can help you improve your performance overall, boost your exercise routine, and restore the body. This could be as easy switching towards organic food and drinks as well more complicated than using cryotherapy for resetting your cellular system. There's no idea how to start. It's best to keep it simple. In the most recent Library of Pursuits course, one of the most effective ways to come up with a strategy is to establish the goals you want to achieve and customize your biohacking strategies to assist you in achieving these goals. Make use of techniques that compliment your lifestyle. These will be easy to learn adhere to, and provide you with the confidence that you can continue to improve your lifestyle. Also, making sure you're eating appropriate proportions of protein carbohydrates, fiber, as well as saturated fats, is equally crucial. Everyone would love to have powers that let us take a flight to work instead using the bus, gaze into the future in order to pick the most lucrative lottery numbers and be able to read minds so that we understand what our coworkers think however the truth is that there are certain items that simply aren't within our comprehension. Even though we don't have the capability to fly as Superman or fire webs from our fingers as Spider-Man (as many as we'd like) We do have amazing capabilities. Human extraction is a distinct characteristic.

The first thing to note is that humans truly possess an incredible quantity of physical strength. It is true that we possess the muscles that are strong enough to slam through the walls, however our brains hinder us from continuously displaying our extraordinary ability. Instead, we reserve all of our potential to the most critical scenarios. Human beings have abilities that are more that physical power. Also, we have a remarkable mental strength. Brains are basically limitless storage devices that are extremely fast computers. Since memory is based on connecting emotional and contextual connections The only reason that our brains aren't able to remember every detail is because of this. The connections diminish if there is nothing that is stimulating them, or they're not strengthened after which the memory becomes "lost" and lost.

There have been instances where individuals are able retain a staggering amount of information either because of obsession or even re-freshing this is as crucial as remembering, since forgetting is the way we set priorities. It's a relief to learn that human beings are also capable of having a pain resistance when all that remembering causes you to get headaches. Humans actually have naturally-occurring painkillers known as "endorphins" that release in the course of physical exercise, extreme pleasure or excitement, or during events that normally cause pain isn't manageable. This is the reason why athletes can perform with pain in competition. Since humans have to experience discomfort to survive Endorphins are a powerful force can't be controlled. Additionally, they direct our body away from harm and devastation.

Finally, use nutrients to boost the quality of your diet. There isn't the nutrients you require through food this is an unfortunate reality of our modern lifestyle. Supplements are available as mineral, vitamins, herbs spice, prebiotics probiotics, as well as postbiotics.

The foundation will be laid by making sure you buy all of them at the amount you need.

Chapter 7: Choose your goal

Being aware of what you are looking for and establishing objectives for yourself are crucial for anyone who is committed to improving your life. Based on Asprey's research most individuals want a combination of these five traits that include increased strength, better endurance, improved cardiovascular fitness and metabolism, enhanced performance of their brains more stress-free, as well as improved recovery.

What is the impact of improved sexual performance, longevity as well as weight loss however? When you figure the remaining five pillars the pillars, they will be "fixed." In addition, as time you will see the four other pillars of the five pillars will change when you build one. The selection of your ideal market is among the initial stages of launching your enterprise. It can be used as a foundation for things that you develop as well as the method by which the company's image is presented and, ultimately, your target audience you choose.You need to create products which appeal to your intended audience with this thought in the mind. Design a corporate website first that embodies your business and incorporates words and imagery that is relatable to the people you are targeting. You should think about the space you are able to fill, and then think about what distinguishes your business apart from competition. As more leads become customers, it is possible to tailor your branding, messaging and marketing specifically to your market.

Find out more about how to identify your ideal market within the following sections Get expert guidance regarding how you can integrate this strategy into the other areas part of your company plan.Your primary customer is the market you want to target. If you can identify the group then you are able to focus your marketing and branding efforts specifically on the people who belong to them. Your target market could be extremely broad, such as married males over 40 in the US as well as very particular for urban, health-conscious vegetarian females in Texas. What needs of the specific customer the product addresses will determine your target market.

The three fundamental elements of a market are listed below:

Demographics, such as income, age, gender degree of education and the status of employment

Geography: The principal location of your store

Personality characteristics include things you like and don't, your preferences for shopping, as well as brands

The analysis of information regarding the product you sell along with your customers and the competition can help determine your market. Furthermore, it is important to be able to better understand your various audiences.

various target markets

Markets targeted by target markets are generally classified in various ways by owners of businesses. Markets targeted by target are typically divided into four types: demographics psychological, geographic and behavior.

1. Demographic:Demographic factors, including age, gender, family size, income, and education, help to determine this type of target market. Based on the demographics of these groups' patterns of spending and purchasing capacity, companies can focus on certain segments of the population.

2. Geographic: Just as the word suggests, geographical characteristics such as areas, states, cities and density of population are utilized to define geographical target groups.

3.Psychographic 4. Psychographic psychological characteristics, such as the way of life, values, personality and socioeconomic background is what defines it.

4. Behavior: The behavior of the consumer which defines this particular type of target market is based on factors like the desire for benefits, use rate, and the level of loyalty. It's important to be aware that based on their specific goals for business and its marketing strategies, companies can select to target one of many categories of markets.

It is crucial to understand the target market. An effective business demands an understanding of your market. The main reasons the need to know your customer's needs for the purpose of creating an effective business are explained in the following paragraphs.

Improved client segmentation Through better segmenting your client base, and understanding your targeted market, you are able to design promotional materials and products which are tailored to the individual's needs and tastes.

Increased concentration and effectiveness by focusing your focus to a specific audience, you will be able to utilize your marketing efforts better and also reduce time and cash by cutting out things that won't be able to reach or connect with the audience you are targeting.

Improved brand image Helping you align your company's beliefs and values of your audience, a thorough awareness of your market helps you create and maintain a solid brand image.

Increased loyalty to your customers by understanding your targeted customer and offering goods and services that satisfy the needs and desires of your customers You can create the foundation of loyal clients that are more likely to recommend your business to other people.

Improved decision-making skills: Understanding the market you want to target will help you make more informed decisions regarding how you design products, determine prices and utilize distribution channels for promotional campaigns.

The term target market and the word "target audience Although they are often used interchangeably they are two distinct terms. The target audience refers to the people whom you promote your product and your market of choice is the ultimate consumer. Though your intended audience might comprise those who belong to your market, the group you select to reach could not necessarily comprise the people who use your product. I'll provide an example for you to understand children are the most evident target audience for kids toy, as an example. It is also a common practice to market toys only to kids that identify with a specific gender. But, parents purchase the toys to their children and not for the kids themselves. To market toys to parents (the the market they are targeting) toys companies need to make sure that their advertisements are targeted at that group.

Chapter 8: Strengthening and improving cardio fitness

A person's fitness and physical strength can be assessed through their endurance to the cardiovascular system. When they add aerobic training in their daily routines, by increasing the intensity as well as duration of their exercise routine everyone of every age will be able to improve their cardiovascular endurance. No matter if you're a child or an older adult the exercise has a variety of benefits for health. The capability of your lungs and heart in their ability to provide you with the oxygen you need while engaging in moderately to intense exercise is known as aerobic fitness. If your cardiovascular health is in good shape, you are able to train for an extended duration at a moderate pace (or brief periods of intense level) before you become fatigued. This can be due to the fact that even while you're exercising your body will keep receiving the oxygen it needs. Your body's ability to move fluids due to your cardio endurance. It also boosts the quantity of oxygen reaching the cells. The muscles' cells and tissues consume the oxygen for the production of energy.

cardiovascular endurance advantages

The improvement in blood cholesterol and blood pressure are just two among the many benefits associated with the endurance of your cardiovascular system.

Helping your life longer and reducing your risk of developing a number of diseases, such as blood vessel and heart problems that can affect your lungs as well as your heart. Aiding you with routine activities (like the lifting of a heavy laundry basket or climbing a flight of stairs) using less effort

Improved mental wellbeing, improved cognitive functioning, as well as general improvement in the quality of living.

Increasing cardiovascular stamina

Training that increases the quantity of oxygen that you breathe could help improve your endurance for cardiovascular exercise. Begin with regular cardiovascular exercises every day for 10-15 minutes. After that, as you increase the amount of time you spend each day, you will gradually increase your physical limits. Adults must be involved in at least 150 minutes exercise per week.

You could increase the length of your walk or increase the difficulty by changing the inclination of the treadmill and increasing the time spent. Each of these can boost your heart's endurance, as well as requiring your body more.A fitness level for a person's physical and aerobic fitness can be determined by their cardiovascular endurance. This is not just for professional athletes. gain from this knowledge.

Someone with strong cardiovascular endurance can often participate in intense exercise for longer time. As performing more vigorous exercise could help to burn off more calories, people looking to lose weight might want to focus in enhancing their cardiorespiratory fitness. Evidence from science suggests positive health effects of increasing heart rate and endurance.

A study conducted at an elementary school the results showed that kids who took part in the sport four times per week, instead of two times per week, increased their cardio endurance. After two to eight weeks of running the endurance of people's cardiovascular system was increased by 4 percent up to 13.5 percentage, according to many research studies. The athletes pushed themselves for between 10 and 30 minutes three times per week. They ran it between three and seven times. They rested for up to 5 minutes between sprints.

The endurance of your cardiovascular system is vital to overall health and goes well beyond race day. According to Sims the best way to think about it is to consider it the basis of the fitness pyramid. The endurance of your cardiovascular system is also a key factor. many potential advantages, ranging from making things a lot easier, for avoiding illnesses. Intrigued? I was too. The best techniques to increase your cardiovascular endurance, how to evaluate them, and the amazing advantages you'll experience both in and outside of the gym are all covered here by professionals.Consider what occurs in the body while you exercise to further deconstruct it. Sims states that after you start exercise the heart rate increases in order to permit more blood to be pumped to the proper regions, specifically your active muscles as well as your skin (to get rid of the heat that your muscles are producing) and away from your organs that are not needed and the digestive system. Elimination of waste as well as the delivery of oxygen for the production of energy aerobically are just two of the things circulation of blood does to your muscles, she adds.

There comes an area where you'll need to stop and recover. With practice, however it is possible to keep your speed for longer, before it occurs. Why? According to Sims one explanation is that the heart has become more robust and the cardiovascularization (number of blood vessels) has grown and this is the reason for the increased endurance of your cardiovascular system. This means that your heart's ability to efficiently pump blood and this means the blood will travel faster. It's easy to say this over and over Imagine being able finish two consecutive Peloton classes, play the entire game of rec league and then lead your group for a long excursion as an example of how improving your endurance in the cardiovascular department will enable you to work out more frequently. This performance benefit is only the iceberg of the of the iceberg. Are you of the opinion that the only method to develop your cardio fitness is running? Sims states that cross-country skiing and rowing are excellent activities to build endurance for your heart. Also, you should look into cycling, swimming as well as running. According to Sims The stress placed on your body is increased as increased muscle use is involved during exercise. Thus, the need for blood rises with speed and can affect the endurance aspect. The rowing sport is one example of how the body must push blood towards your core your upper, and lower muscles.

Go to the gym, do the weights, run around with some weights, and do more, then take protein shakes in the afternoon to build up your strength and faster. It's true that it works. But, unfortunately, it doesn't work even. Combating your body's natural desire to become lazy is not an effective approach. What then?

Proprioceptors are one type of body sensors. They are located, action and movement sensors are looking for you and help ensure that you don't strain yourself too hard. Unfortunately, they can also cause the brain to believe you're capable of doing more than you really can. They can make you believe that you're less fit and have less strength than you actually are. Therefore, you must discover a method to fool those sensors, and not get hurt.

Here are some tips for achieving this What is "metabolic equivalents" (METs) is used to describe the amount of energy that is used in physical activities compared to the energy consumed in the rest of your body. Calculating the amount of oxygen that required by a body when it is at rest is crucial for determining their metabolic equivalents. Get started by using cables, weights, or Nautilus-style gadgets. By using large weights in a proper posture, focus on fast exhaustion. The weights should come down to a minimum of five minutes. Keep doing repetitions till you're exhausted.

Then, do isometric exercises such as holding a plank. While you may not see immediate outcomes, they are effective in the event that you use them briefly.Use resistance bands to perform more difficult exercise too. When you use them, your muscles are likely to fatigue more rapidly. The result? When you lift weights, your muscles are caused to grow 3 times faster.

You shouldn't just rely on the treadmill or exercise bikes to do your cardiovascular workouts! But, these may be better than performing nothing. Get started with interval training at different intensities rather than. Just push or run for about a minute and then slowly lower your intensity to a low intensity for about a couple of minutes. Repeat the exercise for 4 to 5 minutes, stopping whenever your heart rate has reached that level when you started your exercise. The measure of endurance for cardiorespiratory function is the endurance of the lungs, heart and muscles in intense to moderate physical activities. The endurance of the cardiorespiratory system can be increased through regular fitness, specifically the aerobic workout. Aerobic exercise improves the body's capacity to move and use oxygen and improve the health of your lungs and heart.

Consider high intensity interval training as the more difficult exercises. For the first time, head to the park, and walk slow. After that, sprint for 30 seconds in a high speed. When your heart rate is been stabilized, return to your slower walking. Then, another run for 30 seconds. This should last for 20 minutes. When you walk, do meditation. Instead of jogging at a slower pace and jogging, you may want to sit down on the floor to ensure that your heart doesn't need to be working as hard to return blood to your legs.Your fitness level can increase regardless of age. For a better cardiovascular endurance seek the help of a health expert. You will feel more relaxed and the daily tasks can be completed more efficiently. In order to achieve the greatest results begin slowly and keep going. At whatever the stage in your fitness journey you're in cardio endurance is an essential component of fitness. In your own way or in conjunction in the hands of a professional there are many options to develop this and measure the progress you make.

Chapter 9: It is possible to increase the amount of energy you have and your metabolism

Your body creates energy through making air and food into electrical energy. Strength will grow when you become more proficient at it. Your cardio fitness will increase too. The software MeatOS needs to be convinced that you're struggling to enable you to experience increased level of energy. In this case it increases the frequency of mitophagy that removes mitochondria that are weak and not effective, and mitogenesis which generates new mitochondria, which are the "powerhouses that power your cells" increase within the body. Take note of the following: Vibration-based strategies are a great way to begin. The parts of your body that usually receive low levels of oxygen are being re-oxygenated through whole-body vibration. The body is also tricked to believe it's working harder that it actually is. Do something very basic initially, such as vibrating your vocal chords. Vibrations can cause your whole body to sound. Take a seat, breathe an exhale, then say, "Ommmm." It is made more enjoyable through the rebounding. Rebounders are mini trampolines that it is possible to bounce between the ground and up to stretch the body's tissues. In addition and applying spots of vibration that can be extremely damaging to your nervous system as well as accelerate the healing process.

The term"metabolism" describes the whole range of chemical reactions that occur within every body cell and generate energy for the organism. The process of synthesis for new organic materials is fueled by this energy source, and so do vital processes. Each living thing depends on the substances and nutrients present in its environment for its ability to expand, move around, develop, and reproduce. That's how they survive. Each of these steps is executed by the work of enzymes. They are proteins that have specific functions in catabolism as well as anabolism. The metabolic rate of the basal that is affected by factors such as sex or race, physical activity, diet, age, as well as diseases like cancer or sepsis is the pace that energy production occurs.

Every chemical process within your body that help keep you healthy and active are collectively known as metabolic. The metabolism also is involved in transforming substances in food you consume into energy. For breathing and move around and digest food, move blood and repair injured cells and tissues your body requires energy. The word "metabolism" is commonly utilized to describe the rate of your metabolic basal, that is, the quantity of calories that you consume in a state of still. The greater the metabolic rate, the greater number of the calories you consume in still. It is possible to burn off calories while you're sleeping due to fundamental body functions like breathing and circulation, as well as the processing of nutrients and the creation of cells. Age, diet as well as sex, your body's size as well as your health status are just some elements that can alter the rate at which you burn calories. The fundamental metabolic rate defines what this means. The term "fundamental metabolic rate" as well as resting metabolic rate commonly employed in conjunction.

RMR Also known as the resting expenditure of energy (REE) is the number of calories the body burns when it's at rest while BMR is the minimum amount of calories that are required to perform basic processes that take place when you are at rest.

While the fundamental metabolic value and RMR do not have the same degree of consistency however the RMR should be an accurate gauge that you have BMR. They usually diverge in the range of approximately.

Participate actively in improving your health and fitness by being aware of your BMR as well as your normal intensity of exercise, as well as how many calories you'll need every daily to sustain your weight. Knowing your BMR is a great way to decide if you're looking to increase your weight, keep your weight or shed weight. If you have a slow metabolism usually have a higher amount of calories that are stored in fat. The metabolism of your body is the engine that allows you to live. People who have a fast metabolism do however consume more calories, and tend to lose many pounds of weight. Every person is different in their rate of speed.

Calorie consumption and metabolic rate can be described in similar concepts. The body is able to burn a certain quantity of calories within some period of time.

Many evidence-based strategies are able to help you boost the metabolism and help you maintain a healthy weight.

Here are five quick ways to increase your metabolism

1. Every time you eat, take plenty of protein.

The ability to speed up your metabolism for several hours through eating.

Thermic effects of food, also known as TEF is the reason the cause of this. Extra calories that are required to absorb, digest and absorb all the nutrients you consume can be the reason. Protein is the food item that enhances TEF by the highest. Protein from diets requires between 20 and 30 percent of its energy that can be utilized for metabolism in contrast to 5% to 10% in carbohydrates, and between 0% and 3% in fats. Consuming protein has proved to create an immense feeling of fullness, and prevent you from eating too much. Consuming more protein may also help to reduce the decline in metabolic rate that is often associated with weight loss. Protein is responsible for its capacity to prevent losing muscle, which is an often-reported consequence of dieting. With the advancements in body fat control, high-protein diets have been touted as an effective method to reduce or cure overweight for over twenty years. The modulation of the energy metabolism, appetite, and intake of energy are believed to be a factor in these advantages in a way. Protein-rich diets have also been backed through recent studies to reduce cardiovascular risk factors. This article presents a brief summary of recent research regarding the effects on health of longer-term, high-protein diets on the clinical outcome and effects of the consumption of protein in a short period. Numerous meta-analyses of smaller-scale, strictly controlled eating research revealed that more protein-based energy restriction diets led to more weight loss and fat loss and retention of lean mass over low protein energy-restriction diets. Additionally, we observed reductions in the waist circumference, blood pressure as well as the triglycerides. Furthermore, a review of studies on acute eating suggests a slight satiety effect that includes increased levels of levels of satiety hormones as well as a greater feeling of fullness after higher protein meals, however it doesn't suggest a relationship to the caloric intake time of the next meal. An analysis of a recent meta-analysis showed that there are enduring benefits to a high-protein diet to lose weight and fat mass. This is despite the fact that, while short-term and strictly controlled studies of food intake generally found benefits associated with higher intake of protein. However, more long-term studies yielded mixed conclusions. Weight-loss benefits was observed for those who followed the higher protein plan, but those who were not adhering to the regimen did not show substantial advantages. The results suggest that diet compliance can be the major factor leading to these inconsistent results. Together, these findings indicate that high-protein diets generally comprise approximately 1.2 to 1.6 grams of protein per kilogram of body weight each day, but may also incorporate meals-specific amounts of protein that are minimum 25-30 grams for each meal, may increase appetite, body weight management, risk factors for cardiometabolic health as well as all of these results for health. But, further strategies to increase the compliance of a diet for long-term interventions in dietary habits remain needed.

Intensifying your intake of protein can boost your metabolism and aid in helping to burn off more calories. In addition, it aids in improving your feelings of fullness, and also prevent the temptation to eat too much.

2. Drink more water.

Water drinkers who opt for water instead of sugary drinks often experience greater results in losing weight and maintaining the weight off. The reason is that replacing the sugary drink with water automatically decreases the amount of calories you consume since sweet drinks are loaded with calories. The idea has been put forth that drinking more fluids will aid in losing weight however, there's no evidence that this is true. The purpose of this research was to comprehensively review the majority of clinical trials randomized to control for assessed the effect of drinking water in weight, with a time-frame that was at least twelve weeks. In order to locate relevant studies that quantified the body's changes in weight following treatments and treatments, a comprehensive query-based study of PubMed, EBSCO, and the Cochrane Library was conducted. The study included six RCTs which reported a variety of strategies for losing weight, like increasing daily intake of water by substituting water for calorific-rich drinks, as well as premeal waterload. Effects of weight loss after follow-up studies were similar throughout all studies, and ranged between -0.4 kg from -8.8 kg with an average percentage of weight loss being 5.15 percentage. Research showed that shifting between caloric drinks and water is the most effective approach. The amount of evidence that supports the principal outcome in weight reduction was rated as moderate or low. The brief follow-up time is the main negative aspect. Conclusion: Although there an increase of 5.15 percent weight loss the poor to average level of evidence as well as the limited duration of monitoring are limiting the power of suggestions to drink water in order to shed weight. But, it is possible to see an immediate increase in metabolic rate in the event you consume water. This study is a brief advancement of the notion that increased water consumption causes weight loss, primarily due to a decrease in food intake, as well as the loss of fat through increased lipolysis. The research studies cited in these research involve animals, mostly rodents. The research involves alterations of peripheral or central Renin-angiotensin system that enhance drink-related responses while also reducing the body's weight. The theory is based on a general relationship with hyperhydration that is chronic (extracellular dehydration) as well as elevated concentrations of hormone called angiotensin II (AngII) that is linked to various chronic diseases that include diabetes, obesity, cancer, as well as heart disease. A rise in metabolism caused by hydration-induced cell volume growth is among the theories proposed for the effects. Studies that have found these effects usually have human-related applications. Human research supports this notion regarding weight loss, and also reducing the risk factors of being diagnosed with type 2 diabetes as well as overweight. A reduction in eating habits and increased lipolysis are the two main ways by the consumption of more water can be linked with weight reduction. Also, it appears that opposites are true. The weight gain and the related dysfunctions are associated with moderate but constant hypohydration. Angiotensin II (AngII) which is the primary hormone responsible for regulating the body's fluids, is likely to be the most common cause. Evidence is compared with this idea in the following paragraphs.

The study was small and found that drinking 17 8 ounces (500 milliliters) of water over an hour increased resting metabolism by 30%. However, further evidence is needed to prove this in a review from 2013. It can also help provide you with energy if you're looking to shed weight. An analysis from 2015 revealed that drinking water doesn't always lead to an increase in metabolic rate afterward. Based on research that suggest drinking water for 30 minutes prior to eating can help reduce your appetite. Incredibly, one study showed that those who consumed 17 pounds (500 milliliters) of water for 30 minutes prior to meals for a total of 12 weeks, lost nearly 3lbs (1.3 kilograms) more pounds than those who didn't. Weight loss can be reduced and maintain it with the help of drinking water. The water makes you feel fuller after meals and, for a short time, boosts the metabolism.

3. Perform a strenuous fitness routine.

The exercise that's performed by short, quick bursts is referred to as high intensity interval training (HIIT).

It is possible to burn off more fat through a rise in your metabolism when this type of workout will be safe for you to do, regardless of when your exercise has ended. The resistance to insulin (IR) is among the metabolic modifications that are related to the body fat which characterizes overweight. Aerobic exercise, for example intense interval training (HIIT) is among the strategies that do not require drugs to boost the sensitivity of insulin. The study examined the way that eight weeks of HIIT changed both muscle and blood markers to measure the oxidative metabolic process as well as insulin resistance in obese and inactive individuals. It also examined the differences between insulin-resistant and non-insulin-resistant phenotypes.

After 22 hours of moderately intensive and extremely intensive exercise, REE was elevated in energy balancing setting. An increase in sympathetic tone or injury or repair to muscles caused by exercise could be the reason for the increase in REE however, the phosphorylation that is not coupled does not. As per these studies that moderate or vigorous training can increase the amount of energy expended up to 22 hours after exercise.

In comparison to other types of training, this impact could be greater when you do the HIIT. Furthermore, HIIT has been proven to help in losing fat.

This research sought to determine the impact of exercise modes and the pre-exercise carbohydrate, protein, or consumption on the post-exercise energy expenditure and wheezing exchange ratios in females.

A short-term, moderate to high-intensity training for exercise can lead to small improvements in body composition for overweight and obese people with no corresponding body weight changes. Its equal efficacy of MICT and HIIT across every body component metric suggest that HIIT is an efficient and effective component in weight-loss programs.Start with a type of exercise you're already comfortable with, for example biking or running. The metabolism will be increased and fat metabolized through varying the exercise routine by adding a couple of high-intensity exercises.

4. Extra standing

The health of your body may be affected if you are spending too much time at a desk. We don't know for sure what the amount, regularly as well as how much of your inactive time has an impact on results which aren't related to fitness. In order to determine the connection between sedentary time and deaths from all causes, hospitalizations as well as cardiovascular disease as well as cancer, diabetes and all-cause mortality but without considering the physical activities.

The reason is that long time sitting can lead to less caloric consumption and an increase in weight. About a third of the people in the world that are to 89 years old don't exercise enough that has an effect on their overall health. But, it's difficult to know how much health risk sedentary practices present. For the population of adults in Korea it is estimated that sedentary habits last at an average 8.3 hours a day in contrast with 7.7 minutes for Americans. As there are less places for exercise, more people engage in sedentary work things like working from home while television and other video equipment are increasingly utilized and inactive lifestyles are becoming more commonplace across the globe. As a result, problems with health are increasing. Many processes within the human body can be affected due to sedentary living. The activity levels of protein transporters, the muscle glucose metabolic lipids, and carbohydrate metabolism are all affected by the sedentary lifestyle. Also, it reduces the cardiac output as well as blood flow through the body and stimulates the sympathetic nervous system and eventually reducing insulin sensitivity and the function of the vascular system. Furthermore, it affects an insulin-like growth axis as well as testosterone levels in the bloodstream and increases the risk of cancers involving hormones. A lack of activity can lead to an increase in weight, obesity as well as increased chronic inflammation that are all potential risk factors for the development of cancer. Inactivity increases the gravityostat which is the body's homeostat for weight. The wide-ranging negative consequences of sitting down on our body can result in increased mortality from all causes and cardiovascular disease mortality health risks, and risk of metabolic diseases such as diabetes mellitus, hypertension and dyslipidemia. Other conditions of the musculoskeletal system, such as arthritis and osteoporosis, depression as well as cognitive decline. To improve the public's health, it's vital to cut down on sedentary habits and encourage physical activity.

A review of the year 2018 revealed that it was revealed that stepping or standing while working was associated with less triglycerides in the fasting phase as well as the total cholesterol as well as HDL cholesterol levels, insulin levels, the body's weight the waist circumference, diastolic and systolic blood pressure. Standing instead of walking led to greater lower blood pressure in the systolic region as well as insulin resistance.If you are working at a desk, you should consider moving around a bit in order to break your lengthy sitting. Also, you can get a standing desk and consider taking a short walk throughout your time. The prolonged sitting time can cause a loss of calories, and could be damaging for the health of your. Do your best to stand up and walk regularly for walks or purchase the standing desk.

5. Enjoy a glass of Oolong or green tea.

Common tea. It is n. or semi-fermented. It has been demonstrated that they boost metabolism and reduce fat. The caffeine and tea catechins stimulate brown adipose tissues and enhance human thermogenic capability induced by cold. Green tea catechins have been found to exhibit effects on thermogenesis, however the mechanisms behind these effects are not clear.

Teas aid in converting portions of body stored fat into fatty acids that are free that, when mixed together with exercise, could enhance the process of burning fat. The multi-dimensional and complex bodily mechanism that tea helps promote weight loss. In addition the fact that there are many variations in the bioactive ingredients of tea such as catechins, caffeine as well as the byproducts from polyphenol oxidation in tea. Because of its large amounts of phenolic substances and its capacity to sustain the highest levels of antioxidants among any type of major tea green tea has been the primary study of the benefits to health prevention of tea. However, recent studies suggest that the prevention of the accumulation of fat in the body could depend more on antioxidant activity, and more on interactions with gut microbiota as well as enzymes. The aim of this study is to examine the different weight-loss processes due to tea polyphenols and consider what mechanisms are interconnected. According to our initial "short-chain fatty acid (SCFA) hypothesis," the effectiveness of a specific tea for weight loss is affected by both the inhibition of carbohydrate-digesting enzymes and the following interactions of undigested carbs with gut bacteria. These interactions among lingering carbs as well as tea polyphenols and microbes from the colon result in the creation of short-chain fat acids that improve the metabolism of lipids by activating the AMP-activated protein Kinase (AMPK). Based on some studies that oolong, black as well as dark teas that are fermented may trigger the mechanisms that are involved in SCFA synthesizing more powerfully as green teas which did not undergo fermentation. Regarding inhibition of enzymcs and interactions with microbiota in the gut, SCFA synthesis, and lipid metabolism, we have talked about the differences in mechanistic mechanisms between fermented teas and those that are not. This discussion also addresses different outcomes, and the possible cause.

The teas could prove beneficial to reduce weight and maintaining because they're not high in calories. But, research from earlier shows that they don't affect the metabolism. According to research, their effects on metabolism could help people who lose weight to avoid an unavoidable plateau in their weight loss which is caused by slower metabolism. This means that they may not make any effect or be applicable to only a few persons. In a variety of areas around the world, tea has become the most common drink consumed by people. White and green teas are not fermented; Oolong tea is semi-fermented as are black tea and pu-erh tea are fermented completely. Catechins as well as caffeine are major chemical components in teas that are not fermented. arubigins, theaflavins and caffeine are the primary chemical components of semi-fermented and fully fermented tea. The numerous biological effects of catechins and caffeine and theaflavins are well-established.

Prevention of overweight and weight gain is just one of the many functions that these substances are believed to perform. Today, a significant portion of sales in the world comprises "weight-loss teas." But the research relating to the consumption of tea in order to prevent weight gain is complex and constantly evolving. Some studies provide positive results, other studies don't. Green tea was the subject of these studies in the past, as there was a belief that totally as well as partial fermentation of tea polyphenols would not have a significant effect on the weight increase. The assumption might not be correct, based on recent research. Oolong or green tea can boost your metabolism. If weight loss is your aim, these teas may aid, although there is no evidence to support it.

Consuming foods that are spicy can boost the metabolism of your body and aid to maintain a healthy weight. But, they do not have any metabolic boost. The quantity of calories burned, how sugar is processed and the hormones controlling your appetite could all be altered through sleep lack. If you are trying to lose weight as the goal of yours, then drinking coffee is a great way to boost the rate of metabolism. Then, you could offer your MeatOS powerful signals to alter the way it operates by controlling the way you breathe. It is possible to induce controlled hypoxia where the body's system is deprived of oxygen, or thinks it's. The condition can cause death when it is in its worst types. But, if it's under the control of your metabolism, it can perform more efficiently. Just holding your breath can achieve this. Your body's physiology guarantees that you will not become unconscious, thus making it completely safe. Breathing in a controlled manner can trigger angiogenesis, which is the creation of blood vessels that are not yet. Furthermore, it improves the performance of the mitochondria of your body and boosts the flow of blood through a widening of capillaries.Making tiny lifestyle adjustments as well as incorporating these ideas in your routine could help you increase your metabolic rate. If weight loss is your aim, having a better metabolic rate can assist you in doing this while giving you greater energy. These techniques can quickly shift "energy" away from the waistline onto every aspect of your daily routine.

Chapter 10: Increase your senses and skills

If a gorilla first gets confronted with a mirror as scientists have already conducted, it first freezes before thinking, then realizes it is looking at its own reflection. After this, and with a new knowledge of its identity and what it is, it may even begin to snatch leaves that are stuck between its teeth using the mirror for guidance.

What is the significance of this? Your brain's functions are similar to the gorilla. It only has a small perception of its own self due to the fact that the sensors it uses are outside. The brain doesn't think about self-improvement. it simply observes what's taking place within your. However, your brain can adjust, enhance itself, develop, and evolve as long as you can overcome it. Let's take a examine a few ways for doing this:

One option is to utilize a neurofeedback machine at home. These read your brain waves using electroencephalography, or EEG. Through their help it is possible to train your brain to change between different states of mind and to stay composed.Then it is possible to attack your nerves directly especially your vagus nerve which is a part of your brain that travels through the neck to reach the abdomen. The reflex of your body to fight or flee is among its numerous functions. There are many devices that stimulates vagus nerve, which can improve sleep as well as ease migraines and other ailments, decrease anxiety and tension as well as give you a feeling of relaxation and calm.

Many people over the age of 65 put a lot of emphasis exercise for their brains to improve the ability to focus and memory or everyday functioning. It is possible to add a few brain exercises to your routine

routine will benefit people who are of any age. No matter what age you are you can find a number of ways for maintaining your mental acuity. And keep your brain healthy as per studies. You'll be able to perform tasks faster and more enjoyable to perform everyday tasks if you do specific exercises for your brain to increase the quality of your memory, concentration and concentration. The exercises will also assist you in keeping your brain sharp even as you grow older.

We'll take a deeper look at the five activities that provide the most convincing evidence for developing cognitive abilities.

1. Enjoy jigsaw puzzles by playing.

Making a jigsaw can be a great opportunity to sharpen your thinking skills, regardless of whether you're creating a 1000-piece image that depicts the Eiffel

Tower or putting together 100 pieces that form Mickey Mouse.

Jigsaw puzzle solving activates a wide range of brain functions and slows the process of visual cognitive aging, based on research conducted by reliable sources. The process of putting together a puzzle demands you to think about different parts, and then determine what they are in the whole puzzle. The brain is challenged and exercised in a great method by solving this. One of the most difficult to solve medical issues is the prevention of neurocognitive disorders. While it's a common recreational activity for all age categories and a great way to improve your cognitive performance, the benefits from solving jigsaws (JPs) are not previously been examined. Through analyzing the cognitive capabilities that are activated through JP in addition to the advantages to cognitive functioning of an entire and 30-day JP experiences, this research sought to fill the gap between a deficiency of research and a frequent use. Jigsaws, visuospatial cognitive as well as neurocognitive and dementia problems, cognitive aging the cognitive enrichment process, and cognitive intervention and impairment of cognitive function One of the biggest health issues in today's changing society is to avoid the decline in cognitive capacity with age which includes moderate cognitive impairment as well as dementia. Studies conducted on observation have proven that engaging in mentally, physically and socially demanding actions reduces the chance of dementia and cognitive decline. In order to determine the root cause of the observed results, a multitude of random controlled trials of intervention have been carried out. These studies mainly focused on programs for cognitive development such as video games and fitness activities like aerobic exercise as well as resistance training.

Jigsaw puzzles can need a range of cognitive capabilities that include vision (e.g. recognising patterns, objects, and lines orientation) and the constructional praxis (e.g. using both visual and motor inputs for putting the pieces together) as well as the ability to mentally rotate (e.g. the mental rotation of the piece's orientation in order to make it fit with other pieces) as well as cognitive speed and visually scanning (e.g. or sorting puzzle pieces) and also mental flexibility (e.g. changing pieces' orientations to match

In this study, we sought to fill the gap in the absence of studies regarding the cognitive requirements and the effects of jigsaw play and the widespread usage for leisure activities. Puzzles that are jigsaw-like can assist people with stressful situations in calming emotions that is a different elemental component. We first looked into what aspects of the visuospatial brain are utilized when solving JPs. We also investigated by using an observational model to determine whether a the duration of JP exposure is a protective element in visuospatial cognitive decline. Through a randomized, assessor-blinded and controlled study in a clinical setting We examined the impact of a 30 day JP program on the visuospatial memory as the protective factors identified through observational research aren't manipulable and are therefore not cause and effect. Our goal was to find out if there was a correlation between the doses between the amount of solving jigsaws and the JP group's enhancement in visuospatial cognition.

2. Try a few games of cards.

Have you ever had the time you were engaged in playing a game of cards? An hour-long game of cards could boost brain power across a variety of areas of the brain, as per researchers that studied mentally difficult activities for adults. The brain structure of people with Alzheimer's disease preclinically and cognitive function are linked to involvement in mentally stimulating actions.

The game of cards may improve memory and thinking skills According to the same research.

Some of these well-tested and time-tested card games could be worth learning about:

(1) Solitaire A bridge

"gin the rummy" Poker

Heart's

Crazy eights.

3. Expanding your vocabulary

The ability to appear intelligent is with a wide vocabulary. However, did you realize that you could also turn an hour-long lecture on vocabulary into a mental game? A variety of brain regions are involved with vocabulary and language learning as per research findings especially those vital for both auditory and visual processing. The research also shows that the activities associated with vocabulary engage brain regions that were not previously considered. The brain regions that differ in relation to the form of words, like the ventral temporal areas that are important for the use of words in objects that are easily seen as being in close proximity to the places where semantic connections for words are situated. The theory is that ANG and the semantic process work together. The frontal surfaces of the SMG possess a strong connection with the phonological ability. There is a belief that the anterior SMG as well as the ANG are linked by channels that run that connect the SMG's posterior. The left hippocampus as well as the parahippocampal regions are linked to working memory as well as long-term memory and could be a part of the processing of memory that is long-term during vocabulary work. Retrieving phonological information is linked to the precentral structure. Additionally, many more brain structures are related to the vocabulary process, specifically those that process audio and visual information. In addition, the requirements for vocabulary in different languages could cause differences in the anatomy of the brain.

You can try this game to increase your cognitive abilities and confirm the validity of this theory:

Take a notebook with you while you read.

Write down a brand term that is new, and then search it out to find what it translates to. You should try to repeat the word five times during the next day.

4. Make use of each sense.

Involving all the senses could increase your brain's power in accordance with an omnisensory view of working memory. While the vast majority of our sensory perception is multimodal, vast majority of studies on representations of working memory has focused on studying each of the senses individually. The results of the research on multisensory processing suggest that there is more close interplay between our senses than previously believed. These interactions prompt questions regarding how information from multiple sources can be stored in the working memory. The present article examines the situation of research on multisensory processing in the present and examine the implications of these findings for the theoretical knowledge of working memory. To accomplish this, we will focus on studying research in working memory that is conducted using an interdisciplinary perspective and speaking about the relation between attention, working memory to multisensory processing within the perspective of the framework of predictive coding. We believe that the use of multisensory approaches to studying working memory is vital to getting a complete knowledge of how working memory processes manage and store information. We are constantly bombarded with information we experience through hearing, sight or taste as well as touch. As we begin to comprehend the ways that our senses communicate in various phases of processing, it's currently being debated as to whether higher-order mental representations generated by these sensory signals still include specific information about the modality. The reason for this is that, despite the fact that our sensation is mostly multisensory-- that's it is possible to experience information through several senses simultaneously, research in psychology is primarily concerned with investigating our senses as a whole. In particular, studies on working memory has been focused on understanding whether data is stored in discrete specific modality, domain or representations, or in a unified representation.

The interplay of signals that come nearly simultaneously from various sensorimotor modalities are referred to as multisensory processing. In this way, the information received that comes from one mode of perception can affect the way information is processed by the other. Multisensory Integration, a process which combines information from different sensorial modalities into one multisensory experience, is another alternative. In this case, we'll be using the word "multisensory integration."

"Unisensory" also known as "multisensory" is described as a the behavioral or neurological processes that are connected to a particular or a number of sense modalities.

"modality-specific" also known as "cross-modal" is described as the characteristics of objects.

The aim of this research is to analyze the status of research on multisensory processing, and analyze the impact of these findings on the theory of the working memory. This study will examine the research on working memory that was conducted using a multimodal method for this. We will argue that, in order to get an accurate understanding of how working memory is used to save and process information, using a multimodal approach for the research of memory working is necessary.

5.Meditate

It is possible to relax your body and slow down your breathing and let go of anxiety and stress by practicing meditation each day.

There is evidence to suggest that there are numerous benefits of meditation. The research suggests that practicing meditation could aid in improving mood, promote healthy sleep patterns as well as improve the cognitive capabilities of people. The practice of meditation is of educating your mind to concentrate and direct your thought patterns. It's widely known as a way to alleviate anxiety and stress.

With more and more people learning about the numerous benefits it has Meditation is gaining sought-after.

The practice can help you be more conscious about your environment and your own self. It is a method used to develop various healthy behaviors and attitudes, including optimism and a positive outlook discipline, self-discipline and good sleep patterns, and even an improved tolerance to pain. Did you know it could also improve your memory as well as increase the capacity of your brain to absorb data? Each day, you should spend 5 minutes alone while keeping your eyes shut.

The chapter outlines five benefits to health that meditation can bring.

1. Reduces stress

One of the main motives for people to use meditation to ease tension. The study found that the practice did not disappoint in its claim in decreasing stress. In general, physical and mental stress results in increased levels of cortisol stress hormone. Self-care exercises will help reduce anxiety and stress. The result is many negative consequences of stress including release of inflammation chemical compounds known as Cytokines. Stress and anxiety are normal events for many which can be addressed through exercising and meditation. The reality is that millions of people in the US say they experience anxiety and stress on a regular basis.

Everyday stress is a problem for many individuals. It is common for stress levels to be elevated because of factors such as the demands of family life, work as well as health concerns and financial obligations. Additionally, the susceptibility of a person to stress may be affected by many factors that include heredity, level of reinforcement from social networks that they get, their adaption method, and nature of personality. As a result there are some individuals who have a greater sensitivity to stress than other people. To ensure overall wellbeing, it's essential to minimize the constant everyday stress to the maximum extent that is feasible. Stress that is constant affects your health and increases the risk of developing illnesses such as heart diseases, anxiety disorders and depression. It is important to recognize that mental health disorders such as depression or anxiety which require being treated by doctors. Although the advice below will help you deal with a variety of kinds of stress, certain sufferers may not gain from it.

2. reduces anxiety

A meta-analysis of nearly 1300 adults found that meditation can help reduce anxiety. The stress levels are reduced via meditation, and this leads into lower anxiety. A study also found that eight weeks of mindfulness meditation could reduce the symptoms of anxiety of people who suffer from generalized anxiety disorder, as in addition to enhancing positive self-statements and increase stress reactivity as well as the ability to cope. Another research study on 47 individuals suffering from chronic pain discovered that an eight-week mindfulness program brought about significant improvement in anxiety, depression, as well as pain, over an entire year. It is likely to be a consequence of the benefits to health from both physical exercise and meditation.Anxiety caused by job can be alleviated with mindfulness. Based on one study, people who utilized a mindfulness meditation application for 8 weeks experienced higher health, fewer anxiety, and less stress than those who were in the study group. Regular meditation is a great way to reduce anxiety as well as increase the reactivity of stress and the coping mechanisms.We investigated the possibility that a mindfulness-based program available via the smartphone app could enhance the psychological wellbeing of employees, decrease stress at work and decrease blood pressure ambulatory during work. Two38 employees who were healthy from large British companies took part in the study. They were randomly assigned an app for mindfulness practice during for the duration of the study. They were also randomly assigned an app for mindfulness practice for 20 minutes of guided audio meditations. A daily meditation was mandatory for the participants. An additional follow-up questionnaire was sent out to participants at 16 weeks following the time when the treatment started. Blood pressure and psychosocial variables were tracked throughout the work day from baseline to

8 weeks after. Data from usage showed that participants selected randomly for the treatment had 17 on average meditation sessions (range from 0-45 sessions) throughout the eight-week period of intervention. As compared with the group that was a control, participants in the intervention group experienced substantial improvement in their well-being anxiety, stress as well as perceptions of workplace social support. In addition, between the time before and after the intervention, participant's reported blood pressure systolic at work decreased the slightest amount. In the follow-up evaluation after 16 weeks the well-being of employees and their stress were observed to show sustained positive effects for the intervention group. Based on this research that a few short guided meditations regularly on a daily routine could have lasting results on the outcome of the stress of work and well-being. The

short meditations could be accessed via smartphones.

3. Make sure you are taking care of your mental health

Different types of meditation could make people feel more confident at their selves and enjoy an optimistic outlook on living. In one instance, a study of the treatments provided to more than 3500 people found that meditation can reduce effects of depression.Another study revealed that individuals who participated in a mindfulness exercise experienced fewer negative thoughts reaction to seeing images of negative over those who participated in a study group that was not a control. Furthermore, the chemicals that cause inflammation called cytokines can be released when you experience tension, could affect mood. They can also cause depression. according to research from several studies, mindfulness meditation could lower depression levels by reducing the amount of these substances that cause inflammation. The complex mental process of meditation requires adjustments to sensorimotor perception, cognitive autonomic, and hormonal activity. Meditation is commonly used in medical and psychological contexts to reduce anxiety and anxiety-related mental illness, like depression. Many of the physiological systems involved in the pathophysiology behind major depression (MDD) are known to be significantly influenced through meditation, as per the growing amount of research. While improvement in depression symptoms as well as relapse prevention are connected to

The mechanisms that underlie the effects of meditation are not clear and sometimes contradictory. This study examines the causes of a variety of physiological abnormalities that are connected to cytokine activity and

depression mediated by stress in addition to how the various techniques of meditation could be able to help reverse these issues. Certain techniques of meditation can reduce negative thoughts and ease depression. This can also reduce inflammatory the levels of cytokine, which can cause depression to worsen.

4. Self-awareness is increasing:

There is a chance to become your most effective self by engaging in certain types of meditation, gaining more complete understanding of who are.For example, the self-inquiry practice specifically seeks to assist people gain a greater perception of yourself and the way you communicate with your fellow people. Certain types of meditation teach the mind to recognize negative thoughts or even self-defeating.

In theory, through being aware of your thoughts and patterns, you can direct them toward positive patterns.

In a review of 27 research studies, Tai the practice of chi can boost confidence in one's self which is the term which refers to the person's belief in their capabilities or capability to face obstacles.In the study of another, 153 individuals who were using a mindfulness application for a period of two weeks experienced less loneliness and also made more acquaintances over those who were of the group of control. It is also possible that meditation practice can help to develop new ways of solving problems. The effects of meditation in mindfulness on the original thinking is called mindfulness-based creative thinking.

The psycho- and neurocognitive benefits of the mindfulness practice (MM) are been receiving a great deal of interest. Meditation practices like self-inquiry will help you get to "know your self," and can be an inspiration for making various positive changes.

5. could be helpful for overcoming addiction

In a way, you can improve your self-control by increasing your understanding of what can trigger addictive behavior Your mental discipline will gain through meditation could aid in overcoming dependency.

Based on research it is possible to train those who meditate how to redirect on their goals, regulate the impulses and emotions and develop an understanding of the triggers that cause these.

Transcendental meditation has been found to be linked with a lower level of emotional stress, mental distress in addition to alcohol cravings and use of alcohol within three months of a study of

60 individuals receiving treatment for alcohol-related disorders. It can also assist you to manage your food cravings. A meta-analysis of 14 research studies found that mindfulness training helped those who were struggling with emotional eating to control excessive eating. Since treatments for eating disorders and weight loss gain sought-after, mindfulness-based strategies are gaining popularity. While preliminary studies suggest that mindfulness meditation could prove to be an effective treatment for the problem of binge eating, there is no comprehensive review has evaluated treatments in which mindfulness was the principal treatment or at the impact it has on eating or subclinical issues. We reviewed 14 studies that used the PRISMA method for systematic reviews, which looked into mindfulness-based meditations as a primary treatment, and also evaluated the impact of the effects of binge eating,

emotional eating and/or weight loss. The evidence supporting the effects of mindfulness on weight are not all that clear, however it seems to be effective in reducing food cravings and emotional distress in people who engage with these types of behaviors. In order to determine the merits as well as the longer-term benefits of training in mindfulness, further research is needed. It is possible to control the triggers of your impulses through meditation and increasing your mental awareness. It can help in managing unhealthful eating habits and addiction recovery as well as transforming other habits.

The study was conducted over 8 weeks. it was found that the "mindfulness meditation" practice of meditation decreased inflammation triggered from stress.

A variety of different forms of meditation may help to decrease stress. It has been proven that meditation can help alleviate the signs of stress-related diseases like fibromyalgia and post-traumatic stress disorder, as well as IBS. Patients with medical conditions which are made worse by stress could find it helps to feel better. Consider engaging in activities that use the five senses at the same time to work your senses as well as your brain. It might be fun to bake some cookies, visiting a market for farmers, or trying an unfamiliar restaurant while you focus on your senses simultaneously experiencing, smelling, tasting or seeing. Many meditation strategies are a great way to relax and calm your racing thoughts that cause you to stay awake all midnight. The practice of meditation can decrease the sense of pain in the brain, that can accelerate your process of falling asleep and enhance your quality of sleep. If combined with treatment as well as physical therapy it could aid in treating of chronic painful conditions.

In connection with the intimate relationship between your brain and ears Acoustic feedback is an approach to provide specific audio stimulation. Find "binaural beats" on YouTube can allow users to test this feature without cost. It is also beneficial to working on your vision. The practice can help make your eyes sharper. You can try this: keep looking out for the horizon. Try to do this throughout the day but preferably each morning and at night. For at most 3 minutes, look for fifteen seconds at what is happening in front of you and towards the Horizon. The eyes of yours will become stronger and the chance of having visual problems is decreased.

Chapter 11: Reducing your stress levels to enhance the quality of your recovery

The most important thing you can do is decreasing your stress levels. There is a need for a detox not an exercise routine, if you're battling stress. Now let's review of some strategies to reduce stress. It might surprise you by the fact that stress based on biology is not a new idea. Hans Selye, an endocrinologist was not able to recognize or document stress until late in the 1950s. Consider taking a break by listening to calm music if you're overwhelmed by an event that has caused you stress. The soothing music you listen to can have a positive impact on the body and mind as it lowers blood pressure and reduce cortisol, the stress hormone. It is a good idea to take a break from worrying about calling someone you trust and discuss your concerns. Every healthy life requires satiating relationships with family and friends. If you're experiencing a lot of pressure, these interactions are essential. For a short time the soothing sound of a voice could assist you in seeing things clearly. There are times when it is not possible to contact a person. Another option to do in such a situation is to have a conversation with yourself.

Do not worry about being perceived as weird; just talk to yourself the reason you're worried as well as what you need to get accomplished to accomplish the task to be completed, and lastly--that the whole thing will go fine.Dietary practices and stress levels can be interspersed. It is common for us to not take a healthy diet when overwhelmed and resort to unhealthy sweet, salty and sugary snacks to get us going. Make a plan ahead and avoid eating sweet snacks. Vegetables and fruits are generally recommended Studies have proven that fish with a high amount of omega-3 fats can reduce the negative effects of stress. The best brain food for you is tuna sandwiches. The release of endorphins occurs in laughter. They boost the mood, and reduces levels of stress hormones adrenaline and cortisol. Your

the brain's nervous system can be tricked by the brain to create happiness when you smile. It is recommended to see some of the greatest Monty Python sketches, such as "The Ministry of Silly Walking." Then you won't have to laugh anymore since those Brits are hilarious. The consumption of a large amount of caffeine causes an immediate rise in blood pressure. Additionally, it can send your hypothalamic-pituitary-adrenal axis into overdrive. Consider green tea as a alternative to coffee and energy drinks. It is a source of antioxidants that are healthy, theanine, which is an amino acid that helps to calm the nervous system. It also has lower levels of in caffeine than coffee. Also, it has additional nutrients that are beneficial for your health. A majority of the suggestions that we've provided will help you feel better immediately, however there are some lifestyle modifications which may prove effective in the longer term. In recent years, "mindfulness" has gained recognition and is now a major part of contemplative and physical approaches to mental health.

These mindful practices, which include Tai Chi and yoga to Pilates and meditation-- incorporate mental and physical exercises to prevent the stress level from becoming problematic. Consider enrolling in a class. There will be times when you'll experience stress however this doesn't mean you need to avoid the issue. If stress isn't addressed, it can become the most likely cause of dangerous mental and physical illnesses. However, the good news is stress can be reduced. It is possible to lessen stress no matter if it's from the work environment or your family commitments, through a bit of perseverance and some helpful strategies. We could all need a little less stress throughout our lives. There's plenty of stress in the world in the midst of work-related stress and relationship stress. anxiety about social interaction as well as stress that comes with the management of kids. In the event that you put your thoughts to the task, you can find ways for managing stress.

What exactly is stress?

The body is stressed because of the demands or tasks. Everyone experiences moments of stress. These is caused due to a range of causes including minor issues or life-altering events such as separation or loss of employment. An increase in blood pressure and heart rate are signs of stress. They also include thoughts and feelings regarding the event that is stressful and emotion like anxiety and fear.

"Stress is often the result of major lifestyle changes, for example, obtaining a new position at work, or the birth of a baby," explains Dr. Borland. "Although people generally view it as a negative thing but stress may also stem due to unpleasant events within your own lifestyle. People may take a drink or eat a lot in attempts to reduce tension. Short-term the actions may seem to relieve stress, however they can actually cause more difficult. The effects of stress can be made worse due to caffeine. Although a healthy, balanced diet may help in relieving stress, smokers typically refer to nicotine as the best stress relief. Since nicotine can increase the physical arousal, while reducing the flow of blood and respiration and causing more strain on the body. It's not a good idea to smoke if you suffer from constant stress or pain because it could cause chronic pain to get worse. If you're like many individuals, you might find that you're juggling too many tasks to attend to and you don't have enough time within your daily routine. The requirements we face are usually ones that we've chosen. However, you can make better time with time-management strategies such as prioritizing, setting goals and planning time to take care of yourself. The techniques include seeking help whenever needed. No matter how busy your schedule is, you'll be happier when you live your life in line to your beliefs. Before you decide what to accomplish, take into consideration your dreams.

The Dr. Borland advises that we must pursue interests that align with our ideals and communicate about ourselves personally in context of the demands and pressures that we have to face each day.

The ability to say "no" to time and commitments to energy that place your life under stress can be normal. It's not necessary to conform the expectations of others.

When we break during the course of the day anxiety anxieties, worry and tension can be lessened. We often do not stop. It is possible to improve your mental wellbeing in only 10 minutes. It's time to commit ourselves an hour this morning to be kind to our own well-being. Stress can aid to accomplish things as stress is a normal element of life. In fact, stress levels above the normal could be an inevitable element of daily life, especially in the following of a trauma such as a major illness such as a loss of employment, the loss of a loved one in the family, or another difficult situations. There is a common tendency to experience anxiety or depression during a time.

See your physician if you suffer from anxiety or depression longer than several weeks, or when it begins to impact your activities at home, or at workplace. Some other methods, including therapies and medicines, may help helpful.Being in a stressful situation can assist in completing tasks as stress is an inevitable part of human life. Stress levels that are high are a common element of daily life following a trauma or a serious illness or job loss an untimely death in the family or in other stressful situations. You may experience anxiety or depression at times. See your doctor if are experiencing anxiety or depression longer than several weeks, or when it begins becoming a problem for you either at home or at work.

These suggestions could prove helpful in reducing stress

Maintain a cheerful outlook.

Try to be assertive rather than violent. Instead of being frustrated, defensive or smug, speak your feelings, thoughts, or beliefs.

Improve your time management skills.

Set reasonable limits and decline any requests that could put excessive stress on your daily life.

Give yourself time for your passions and interests.

Beware of using substances such as alcohol, drug use, or addictive habits in order to ease tension. Your body can experience increased anxiety if you take alcohol or drugs. Get involved in social interaction. Spend time with your loved ones enough time.

To find more nutritious methods to manage pressures in your life get assistance from a psychologist or another mental health professional with expertise in stress management or biofeedback methods. The way you feel is significantly affected by the way you react to the stress. The blood tension, blood sugar and various bodily functions could be benefited. For a reduction in tension now make use of these techniques to relax. There is always stress. From small annoyances to more serious issues. Although you cannot always alter the circumstances around you, you can determine how you take a stand. The health of your body can be affected in the event that stress becomes extreme or persists. This is why using effective stress relief products which can relax your mind and body is vital.

One of the most efficient techniques for reducing stress are:

Meditation, guided imagery or progressive relaxation of muscles, breathing deeply, going for an afternoon walk, giving hugs as well as aromatherapy. A healthy diet, medications for stress relief or pastimes, constructive self-talk, yoga, gratefulness and exercise, focusing, relationships, and reduction of stressors are but a few methods to lessen stress.But in the case of the reduction of stress, there's not an all-encompassing solution. Whatever purpose one person has might not work for another. Additionally, what is effective in your home environment may not be a viable option for you when working or out and about (dancing in your living space may be beneficial, but dancing outside the store may not be.).

It's essential to have several ways to manage stress available to help manage stress. In the end, you'll have to choose the method most suitable to your particular circumstance the best.

Quick-Relief Techniques for Stress

What techniques quickly reduce stress? Meditation and deep breathing are two effective practices are practiced at any time any time, and at any location, to achieve immediate outcomes.

It is essential to keep stress-management techniques in place to lessen your stress as soon as possible regardless of whether you're preparing going to an interview for a job or are being overwhelmed by your child's behaviour on the playground.

A good short-term strategy is:

It is easy to master, is completed anywhere, costs nothing and gives rapid relief.

In addition to immediate stress reduction, the long-term advantages of managing stress come through the practice of meditation. It is possible to experiment with different methods of meditation that are unique and attractive to the individual in their own unique way. Create your own mantra, which you keep in your mind as you take long, steady breaths. Or, you could devote a brief time practicing mindfulness in which you are aware. Focus on the things you are able to hear, taste or feel, as well as smell right now. If you're in the present moment, you're in no position to dwell on the past or fret over the coming days. Though they are not without to be practiced, meditation and mindfulness will significantly lower your stress levels by taking your attention back to the moment. For reducing anxiety, you can use progressive muscle relaxation (PMR) which was initially invented by American doctor Edmund Jacobson in the 1930s is a method of alternating between tensioning and relaxing all one of the muscle groupings. It is likely that your muscles are tight and stiff when you are suffering from anxiety disorders like Social Anxiety Disorder (SAD) as well as generalized anxiety disorder (GAD). Find out how relaxed muscles feel differently than a muscle that is tight when you practice PMR.

Most of the time, the systematic desensitization process and other treatment methods for cognitive behavior that include progressive relaxation, are incorporated. But, doing the method by yourself can give you greater control over the way your body responds to stress.

It is possible to fall asleep when you do this technique effectively. If that is the case, you should be elated on your accomplishment in reaching the state of relaxation. Also, be grateful for your efforts to this level. If you are suffering from any medical issues, talk to your physician prior to beginning the relaxation exercises.Your general stress level could be reduced by just paying close attention to your breathing, or changing the way you breathe. Within a short time breathing exercises can ease your body as well as your mind. What's more, there is no way to be noticed doing the exercises. So, breathing exercises can aid in reducing your anxiety, no matter the situation, whether it's a stressful meeting or in a crowded theater. Just a couple of minutes to get your exercise functioning as a stress relief. It is possible to experience a shift of scenery when walking to help you change the way you look at things as well as provide the health advantages.

Walking is an easy and effective method to refresh your body and mind, regardless of whether you need to stroll in the office for an escape from the monotony of your task or take a long walk at the park following work. Stress can be significantly decreased by touching. The act of hugging your loved ones is a great way to relax. Oxytocin (often known as"cuddle hormone "cuddle hormone") can be released in hugging. More happiness levels as well as less stress levels are connected to the hormone called oxytocin. Apart from lower blood pressure, it can also reduce the stress hormone, norepinephrine, and may create a sense of feelings of calm. If you're in need of to be hugged, don't feel afraid to ask your friend or loved one to give one. It is beneficial to both you and is one of the easiest methods for relaxation that are available. Recent research suggests that certain scents can affect brainwave activity, and decrease levels of stress hormones that are present in our body. Aromatherapy can be extremely beneficial in stress reduction. It can make to feel more relaxed, energetic or even more at your present moment. You can add some scents to your daily routine, no matter if you prefer candles, diffusers or other body products. Perhaps it was easy to access your creativity when you were younger even if you've lost the passion for artwork, there's still the possibility to do it.

If you're not interested in drawing or painting consider coloring books. Coloring books for adults are becoming increasingly well-liked, and with great reason. Coloring is a wonderful means of decompressing.

Studies consistently show the benefits of coloring. Coloring can create an calming effect. In one study the people who colored complex geometric patterns experienced less stress levels. This makes it the best exercise to relieve anxiety. What steps can you make for the longer term to ease stress in your brain? Certain actions can increase resilience to stress as well as improve overall health. For example, people who regularly practice exercises or meditation are less stressed when confronted with a tough situation. So, it's crucial to develop an approach to life which will allow you to manage anxiety and overcome difficulties in a way that is healthy. Poor diets will make you more susceptible to anxiety. Sugary carbs like chips made from potato and cookies could trigger a high blood sugar. The emotional eating habit and the desire to eat the high-fat and high-sugar food group may give you a short-term feeling of relaxation, which can increase your anxiety over the long term. It is possible to feel worried and stressed in the event that your blood sugar falls.

The long-term management of stress is possible by taking a balanced and healthy diet. Energy balance and mood management are aided by foods such as avocados, eggs and walnuts. While many believe that they are too busy to have hobbies, games or any other fun activities, a little having some leisure time can be a great option to lower anxiety. Incorporating time for leisure time within your daily schedule can help ensure that you're always feeling the best. The pursuit of hobbies and entertainment is essential for living your life to the fullest no matter if you feel fulfilled taking care of your garden or love creating quilts. If you're more relaxed and perform better and your you'll have more leisure time. time could make your work time productive. What you say about yourself. Doubts about yourself, self-criticism that is harsh, and doomsday scenarios won't help. It's easy to stress yourself out when you constantly tell yourself "I do not have the time to do that" or "I am not able to endure this." It's important to develop a more realistic and compassionate inner dialogue. Be able to respond to self-talk that is negative and self-doubt by engaging in a compassionate inner dialogue. Because of its apparent positive vibe and accuracy it is believed that happy individuals are happy can appear on a bumper sticker. But research on gratitude supports this notion. There is a feeling of joy to have someone do something nice for you that fills you and fills you with gratitude.

There are also ways you can use your daily life to generate feelings of gratitude yourself and your experiences already have, and also make new ones that give you more joy to your own life, and your loved ones close to you. There is no need to wait around for events to trigger this emotion for you. Many benefits result out of this feeling, one of them is a greater resilience to stress. These are proven ways to increase your gratitude when you interact with people There are simple actions that you could do on your own and get a tiny burst joy, while some are routine practices that boost your mood and provide you with more peace of mind. Some were impressive actions which you'll remember to come back. Think about the suggestions below and find out ways to improve your quality of life by expressing gratitude no matter what it is you want. Whatever the reason you're happy, research has shown that smiling can affect your mood. There are two benefits: You feel more confident in yourself and can be surrounded by the world full of happy, smiling people. In addition, you will notice that people often respond with a smile whenever they observe an actual smile on another's face. If you're facing a difficult situatlon, a smile will quickly sooth a difficult social interaction, and help lower anxiety levels. Journaling can provide many benefits such as improved health and improved resilience. However, there's an added benefit to keeping an appreciation journal. Make a list of three things for that you're grateful every day towards the end of your day (or when you require an energy boost) And really enjoy the positive feelings that come up as you consider these things. There is evidence that keeping a journal of gratitude will help alleviate sadness and reduce anxiety. The well-known loving-kindness practice offers benefits of the practice as well as that increase compassion and relationship. The practice begins with focusing on positive, loving self-esteem and expands from there. It helps you savor the feelings of gratitude you feel for the people who are important that you have in your life, and also in creating more gratitude towards those are difficult to understand. Every person has the capacity to be envious after someone gets a promotion that they believed they would be meant to get, or someone enjoys that "perfect" relationship, or has the amazingly healthy children that they have had always hoped to have and when someone has everything we want (but aren't getting) within our lives. We rarely desire to swap our entire lives for someone else, rather, we would like to have could have that thing is theirs that could make our lives more pleasant. People who suffer from envy usually compare the least desirable things about their lives to the positive qualities that others have. We also compare our most difficult circumstance with someone else's best day and quality or. If you're fighting with the green-eyed monster shifting your perceptions of comparisons and incorporating more gratitude can help escape from the pain. If you find yourself longing for some thing that someone else does then tell yourself to appreciate your own achievements instead of feeling in jealousy of their success. Take note of all the aspects in your life in which you shine and be grateful for them when you feel unworthy due to the fact that a friend does things better than you. The idea is to take pride in your achievements and gratitude for the things you've accomplished to combat the urge to be jealous. These jealousy episodes will quickly transform into a routine and occur much less often. As per research, those who appreciate their surroundings are healthier mentally as well as less stress as well as a more enjoyable living. Develop a habit of gratitude by writing three things you're grateful for every day in a gratitude journal or creating an everyday routine to acknowledge your gratitude with your family around the table for dinner. Eliminating something from your daily routine could be the best relief from stress. For a more peaceful and relaxed feeling eliminate your stress-inducing things. stress you.

A way to add anxiety on your mind is to keep up with the news or be connected to gadgets all the time and drink alcohol or consume a lot of coffee. Perhaps you feel better when you make a few changes in your routine routine. You may need several trials and errors to discover the best methods for relieving stress. Some strategies might require further practice.However you must keep searching for sources that allow you to manage the inevitable ups and downs of life. To maintain your health overall you must manage the stress you feel.

The physical symptoms of stress. Individuals respond to stress in various ways. Changes to appetite or sweating or difficulty sleeping are just a few common symptoms of stress. These signs are caused due to an increase in stress hormones that are present in your body. They release gives you the capability to deal with the pressure or risk. "Fight or flight" response is the one described to explain this. The hormones noradrenaline as well as adrenaline that trigger your heart rate to increase, as well as perspiration production and blood pressure to increase. The body then is prepared to react in the event of an situation of emergency. The hormones also reduce the stomach's activity and slow the flow of blood to the skin. Cortisol, another stress hormone is a stimulant for energy, taking sugar and fat out of the system.

The result could be headaches, nausea, vomiting tension in muscles, pain or disorientation. You may also be breathing more rapidly, feel symptoms of heart palpitations or numerous pains and symptoms. In time it could increase your chance of heart attacks or strokes.These features have been handed through to us humans by the time of our ancestors, that needed to avoid danger or fight. Stress hormone levels usually get back to normal after the stress or threat is gone. But if you're in constant stress the time and you're constantly under stress, the chemical compounds remain within your body, causing signs of stress. It's impossible to use the substances your body makes to protect you when you're in a busy train or office as you're unable to get away from it. The accumulation of these compounds as well as the modifications they trigger with time can be damaging for the health of your body.

The emotional and behavioral effects of stress

In times of stress it is possible to feel a myriad of feelings, including anger, frustration, or low self-esteem. These may cause you to withdraw and rethink, even to cry. You may experience times where your mind is racing and you are constantly worrying or find yourself contemplating the same issues repeatedly. Certain people notice changes in their behavior on their own. Some may act out in an unpredictable manner or lose their temper faster, or increase the physical or verbal anger. These physical manifestations could exacerbate the conditions and make you experience a greater amount of discomfort. In particular, experiencing severe anxiety may cause you to feel sick that you start to worry it could be caused by an illness that is dangerous.

Recognizing the signs of stress

Everybody experiences anxiety. But, it's important to manage the issue as swiftly as is possible when it is affecting on your lifestyle, health or overall wellbeing. While everyone experiences stress in different ways There are a few typical signs and symptoms that you must be aware of

Constant worry or anxiety

Surreal sensations

Problems with concentration

Changes in mood or mood your mood

An excessive amount of irritability or an instant temper

Trouble unwinding

(1) Depression

Low self-esteem

Modifying one's usual eating routine

Changes in sleeping patterns

Involvement with illicit substances such as tobacco, alcohol or alcohol for relief from pain and Aches and stress, particularly in the muscles. It can cause constipation or diarrhea.

Lightheadedness, nausea or vomiting

A decline in the sexual drive

Talk to your physician when you've experienced this type of symptom for a lengthy time and you feel that they affect your daily routine or make you feel unwell.

Get them to provide you with information on solutions and solutions you can access. The signs of stress were present way before Selye was born, but his discoveries led to new research that helped millions of people to manage their anxiety. This is a listing of our top ten stress relief exercises.

The first thing to do is sleep. Why is it that sleep appears all over the place? There's a reason for that. If you're getting enough sleep the body's natural capacity to repair and create new tissue gets better. Make use of blackout curtains, turn off your lights in the evening switch off your electronic devices for at least 2 hours prior to going to sleeping, and increase the brightness of your mobile to aid in greater sleep. Consume nothing but food for at most two hours before you go to go to bed. A daily meditation practice can benefit you. Stress makes it challenging to sleep as it's well acknowledged.

Unfortunately, sleep deprivation is a significant cause of stress. The body and brain are disoriented because of this cycle of stress, and it will only get worse with time.Make sure you get 7 to 8 hours of sleep every night as your physician recommends. Make sure you give your body time to relax before heading to sleep by switching the television off earlier, and dimming your lights. In our top list of calming substances this might be one of the most effective.

The sun's body is able to produce more serotonin as well as vitamin D because of sunlight exposure and boosts the mood. If you want to reap the maximum benefits take a walk at sun's rays in the morning, or even in early after lunch. Asprey suggests spending at the very minimum 15-20 minutes a day applying your face.

Lastly, herbs. For stress relief, try Rhodiola, ginseng and Ashwagandha. They're safe to take regularly for the vast majority of people. But, if you're currently taking any kind of medicine, you should consult with your physician prior to taking any medication.

Finally, saunas. They speed up your recovery as well as allowing the sweating out of the toxins. Beginning by doing five to ten minute sessions. Then, gradually move towards 20-minute saunas 3 times per week.

In short, you can lower stress levels by taking a break and soaking up some sun as well as getting a better night's sleep as well as making use of a sauna.

Chapter 12: Recover the brain you need

Now you know ways to maximize the essential human capabilities that include strength, cardio mental energy and anxiety. A variety of methods and instruments that can help to improve your performance however, if you wish to go higher, you'll need to reenergize your energy. Science, however, suggests that focusing on the basics--food and sleep that nourish your brain may be the ideal option for action.The time following my long ride was among my favourite times of the day in my younger years. After I returned at home, I would make large smoothies, sit down to take a break from an show that I had never admitted I had, then unwind through a long stretch.That long, arduous routine was among the many things that needed to go in when I began managing teams while participating. I continued to stretch however, I was doing other things. The effects soon began to show of this, such as cramping my calves as well as difficulty in getting myself to go on trips. The issue grew into one that lasted throughout my entire training season. it was only when I finally found time to stick with a strict recovery program that my issues could be resolved. There are a variety of techniques and equipment for us to use to speed up recovery and aid in our adaptations to training. These include the non-steroidal anti-inflammatory medications (NSAIDs) such as foam rolling compressing clothes and ice baths. There are also energy replacement, and heat for only a few.Which method is most effective of all? Which should be the main focus on our time? Which one of the methods suggested by science is most effective? Recent reviews of the empirical literature like one that was conducted by the team by Dr. Andrew Peterson, the University of Iowa's director for sports medicine, found no evidence to support the efficiency of a variety of strategies. They could hinder performance under particular circumstances, for example the use of icing when heat is applied as well as when NSAIDs are used.What is it that makes athletes invest such a lot of time and money to use the use of these techniques? According to Dr. Peterson's view is easy: "People want to maximize every aspect of their lives."

After a hard workout, a number of athletes experience a feeling of being uneasy and feel like they must perform something in order to recuperate. However, sometimes staying in the moment is the best way to go. That is allow your body to do the things it was made to accomplish. A majority of currently utilized rehabilitation tools and modalities were studied through the eyes of the Dr. Peterson for his review and found small benefits. Dr. Peterson also believes that the study may have underestimated benefits because of publishing bias and financial conflicts. (Many negative studies have never been published, and if they were published, the results of studies would show lower impact.)

Peterson recognizes that such techniques could be limited to minor improvement. Many people may not be of clinical value but for the grand tour cyclist, they may be significant.One issue is that there's not much money or motivation for studies on recovery to understand the numerous consequences. The research on the recovery of performance racing have revealed that the brain EMG activity is in line with.

Rattray's work focuses on the role of the brain in rehabilitation. Rattray says of current treatment methods for recovering, "I don't know if we're going in the wrong direction." I'm just wondering if we've considered every option."

A majority of research on healing concentrates on the muscle's peripheral areas, an area that all of them have in their common. Yet, Rattray explains that our central nervous system is extensively studied as a major factor in weariness from the beginning of the beginning of the 19th century.

According to Peterson that there's always some amount of neurophysiologic exhaustion. Central governor theories of fatigue is based on the idea that feeling fatigue in a race or tough bike ride might be a result of the brain is accepted as a fact by athletes. The brain tells us to reduce our speed to prevent harm.Rattray has discovered that the central governor could have a hand in recovery too. It could be one of the reasons that drive athletes to use restorative methods which have no effect on repair and recovery of muscles. Potential benefits for mental health. Rehab strategies may are able to create a strong placebo effect, as per Rattray's studies. The re-generation of glycogen in muscles via the consumption of carbohydrates that are simple after competition or training is an accepted method of recovery. An inter-institutional study conducted in 2013 revealed that cold-water bathing stimulated the brain, which has been associated with fatigue during cycling in heat.Cycling According to Rattray "is all about getting energy back to me." Motivation is a high-energy task for the brain. Moreover, the feeling of fatigue has been shown to reduce the time to exhaustion while on cycling. We've probably not thought about the fact that our brain also requires fuel. Also physical exhaustion could cause severe signs of mental fatigue. According to Rattray the brain's power is exhausted, "you lose your ability to keep going, and then you'll quit. "Following the demands of a rigorous workout the athletes must recharge their energy. The consumption of food and other nutrients play part in the replenishment process in certain instances. Rattray also says that it's about relaxing the brain. The most current developments in the field of recovery may require us to go back to earlier methods.

"I believe that a large part of recovery really comes down to the food you consume every day as well as the sleep that you're getting." Peterson asserts.

It is possible to try compression tights or submersion in the cold water. You could avoid a gruelling recovering process that can create anxiety, keep it simple and stay with the fundamentals. It's better to rest according to Peterson He is even more direct in his explanation.

Conscious healing

Instead of following the research suggests, many athletes have developed their own regimens of recovery by trial and failure. Here are some tips from our professional athletes if looking for help in making your own.

Don't interfere with your process of the body's natural processes.

According to Peterson the evolution of life has created many extremely intricate methods of recovery. It has a fantastic job in repairing itself. It is all you have to do is step away from the way.

Educate your mind.

Rattray believes that we can build our mental resiliency just like regularly exercising on bikes can increase the endurance of our body. Consider using some applications for brain training when

.

cycling in the winter. "Even taking part in activities that stimulate your brain when you're doing your exercise is an option that has been proven to be quite beneficial in its results."

Switch off and disconnect from the brain.

Removing yourself from the world of technology and stimuli is among the easiest ways to recover, at the very least, in theory. Instead, build relationships with your friends and concentrate upon activities that bring your joy.

Rattray claims that in a scientific sense it helps to refill the brain's supply of fuel. He suggests against tasks that are mentally demanding, pointing out that emotional stress is particularly depleting. Activities that help to calm your mind and aid in healing are going to the movies and hanging out with buddies, or relaxing and enjoying music.

relax and drift off

The new recovery you've been looking forward to after a bicycle ride may simply be an hour-long sleep. Rattray claims that when we sleep our brains replenish their reserves of energy. Peterson claims that in the same time that our muscles heal themselves. Peterson asserts that an injured athlete should not sleep in excess.

One of the most effective recovery methods you could employ is replenishing glycogen levels in your muscles as well as the brain. It is recommended that the American College of Sports Medicine suggests taking 1.2 up to 1.5 grams of protein for each kilogram of body weight immediately following exercise. And, the sooner you start eating the more beneficial. According to Peterson that your body's capacity to replenish glycogen storage more rapidly when you begin to consume carbs.

www.ingramcontent.com/pod-product-compliance
Lightning Source LLC
Chambersburg PA
CBHW051726020426
42333CB00014B/1176